Besma HAMDI
Sabrine Louhaichi
Agnès Hamzaoui

Adolescent asthma

Besma HAMDI
Sabrine Louhaichi
Agnès Hamzaoui

Adolescent asthma

ScienciaScripts

Imprint

Any brand names and product names mentioned in this book are subject to trademark, brand or patent protection and are trademarks or registered trademarks of their respective holders. The use of brand names, product names, common names, trade names, product descriptions etc. even without a particular marking in this work is in no way to be construed to mean that such names may be regarded as unrestricted in respect of trademark and brand protection legislation and could thus be used by anyone.

Cover image: www.ingimage.com

This book is a translation from the original published under ISBN 978-620-6-72351-6.

Publisher:
Sciencia Scripts
is a trademark of
Dodo Books Indian Ocean Ltd. and OmniScriptum S.R.L publishing group

120 High Road, East Finchley, London, N2 9ED, United Kingdom
Str. Armeneasca 28/1, office 1, Chisinau MD-2012, Republic of Moldova, Europe
Printed at: see last page
ISBN: 978-620-8-14315-2

TABLE OF CONTENTS

INTRODUCTION

Asthma is the most common chronic disease affecting adolescents. According to the ISAAC study (International Study of Asthma and Allergies in Childhood) [1], the overall prevalence of asthma in the 13-14 age group is estimated at 13.7%, with significant variation between countries around the world. Tunisia is one of the high-prevalence countries.

Adolescence is a period of transition from childhood to adulthood. It is characterised by profound physical, emotional, intellectual and psychosocial changes.

Teenagers have the task of becoming familiar with their growing bodies, acquiring a degree of independence from their parents, developing their own network of relationships and making important decisions about their education and future.

Having a chronic illness, such as asthma, at this age will hinder the adolescent's process of autonomy by reinforcing their dependence on their parents. What's more, the restrictions and therapeutic constraints of the disease will work against the need for emancipation and experimentation that are necessary to the process of building one's own identity.

Adolescence is a high-risk period marked by denial of the disease, poor adherence to treatment and risky behaviour [2].

Asthma control is a concept which refers to the evolution of the disease over a period of a few weeks [3]. It reflects the extent to which the disease is controlled by the management provided, and therefore reflects the activity and dynamic nature of asthma over a given period, regardless of its severity [4].

During adolescence, asthma is often poorly controlled [5,6], with a substantial impact on quality of life and schooling [5] and a high economic cost [6]. For these reasons, asthma control is considered to be the main objective of asthma management according to international recommendations [7].

The aims of our study were to investigate the clinical, functional and therapeutic features of adolescent asthma and to identify factors influencing disease control.

PATIENTS & METHODS

A. Study framework :

This study was conducted in the Paediatric Pneumology B department of the Abderrahmane Mami Hospital in Ariana. It was a cross-sectional and descriptive study with retrospective data collection over a 5-year period (2015-2019). Fifty adolescents were included and divided into two groups according to the level of control: a controlled group and an uncontrolled group.

B. Patients :

I. Inclusion criteria :

We included in this study all adolescents aged 10 to 19 years who were hospitalised in the Paediatric Pneumology B department of the Abderrahmane Mami Hospital in Ariana, or seen on an outpatient basis between January 2015 and June 2019 for asthma.According to the WHO, adolescence begins with the onset of physiologically normal puberty and ends when adult identity and behaviour are accepted. This period of development corresponds to the period between the ages of 10 and 19 [8].Asthma is defined according to GINA 2018 by a history of respiratory symptoms such as wheezing, breathlessness, chest tightness and cough that vary in time and intensity and are associated with variable expiratory flow limitation [7].

II. Non-inclusion criteria :

Not included are :

*Children with chronic obstructive pulmonary disease of other causes and congenital heart disease.

*Children under the age of 10.

III. Exclusion criteria :

We excluded patients with incomplete records.

C. Methods :

I. Control level :

The level of asthma control was specified according to the levels defined by the Global Initiative For Asthma (GINA) 2018 (Appendix 1). The level of control during the last consultation was used.

II. Data collection :

Data were collected from medical records and outpatient consultation forms and recorded on an individual form (appendix 2). La form a included different variables concerning the epidemiological, clinical, functional and therapeutic characteristics of patients.

Epidemiological characteristics :

We noted :

*   Age at inclusion

*   Sex

*   Weight

*   Smoking (passive and active)

*   Socio-economic conditions

2. Clinical features :

We noted :

*   Age at onset and diagnosis of the disease.

*   How long the disease progresses.

*   Associated atopic symptoms (allergic rhinitis or conjunctivitis and atopic dermatitis).

*   Family history of atopy and asthma.

*   Associated co-morbidities (gastro-oesophageal reflux disease, overweight and obesity).

Overweight and obesity are defined as a BMI above the $85^{\text{ème}}$ and $95^{\text{ème}}$ percentile respectively, according to the CDC curves (appendix 3).

3. Characteristics of asthma :

*   **Allergic nature:** the allergological skin investigation was based on a meticulous and detailed questioning, supplemented by the Prick-Test technique.

The allergic nature of the asthma was determined on the basis of positive skin tests for pneumallergens. The allergens tested were house dust mites: Dermatophagoides pteronyssinus (DP) and Dermatophagoides Farinae (DF), cat hair, dog hair, 5 grasses, olive, cypress, parietaria, cockroaches and feathers.

*   **Control of the disease during the last four weeks :**

- The frequency of use of bronchodilators.

- The frequency of nocturnal and diurnal symptoms.

- Limiting activity because of his asthma.

The level of disease control was assessed by reference to GINA 2018 (Appendix 1).

* **Asthma severity:** can be assessed when the patient has been on regular background treatment for several months [7] :

- Mild asthma: this is asthma that is well controlled by treatment levels 1 or 2.

- Moderate asthma: this is asthma that is well controlled by level 3 treatment.

- Severe asthma: this is asthma which requires treatment levels 4 or 5 to be well controlled, or which remains uncontrolled despite treatment (appendix 5).

* **Disease profile over the last 12 months :**

- The number and severity of exacerbations.

- The number of emergency consultations.

- The number of hospital admissions.

- Limitations to physical effort.

- Truancy.

4. Psychological assessment :

It was carried out by the department's psychologist by means of an interview with the patients accompanied by their parents.

5. Respiratory function :

- The peak expiratory flow (PEF) recorded at the last consultation was recorded. PEF was assessed according to the patient's height (appendix 6).

- Respiratory function tests (RFT) were performed using spirometry. Values for forced expiratory volume in one second (FEV1), forced vital capacity (FVC) and Tiffeneau index were recorded. A bronchodilator test was used to assess the reversibility of the obstruction. The relevant ventilatory parameter was measured again after inhalation of 400 µg of salbutamol.

The result of the last spirometry was used: normal (FEV1 normal and Tiffeneau index > 90%), reversible obstructive syndrome (Tiffeneau index < 90% and 12% reversibility of FEV1 compared with the reference value).

6. Biological investigations :

We raised the :

*Level of eosinophils in the blood.

*Determination of total IgE antibodies.

7. Therapeutic characteristics :

* Background treatment: inhaled corticosteroids (ICS), long-acting beta-2 mimetics (LABMs) and antileukotrienes.

For each drug, we have specified the name of the molecule, its dose and route of administration.

* The inhalation technique used: device used (metered dose inhaler (MDI) with or without inhalation chamber (IC), dry powder inhaler) and the quality of the inhalation technique.

* Therapeutic compliance: good or poor (assessed on the basis of compliance with doses and the number of times the asthma medication is taken).

III. Identification of groups :

According to GINA 2018 [7], 50 adolescents with asthma were divided into two groups: a controlled group of 28 patients and an uncontrolled group of 22 patients.

The epidemiological, clinical, spirometric and therapeutic characteristics of each group were specified and compared.

IV. Definitions :

1. Asthma attacks :

It is a brief paroxysmal attack of dyspnoea, chest tightness, wheezing or cough, which subsides spontaneously or with appropriate treatment [9].

2. Asthmatic exacerbation :

The persistence of respiratory symptoms lasting longer than 24 hours, regardless of whether the onset is gradual or abrupt, and requiring a change in treatment [9].

V. Statistical analysis :

The data were analysed using SPSS version 17 software.

1. Descriptive study: we calculated absolute frequencies and relative frequencies (percentages) for the qualitative variables. We calculated means, medians and standard deviations and determined extreme values for quantitative variables.

2. Analytical study: comparisons of two means on independent series were carried out using the Student's t-test.

Comparisons of percentages on independent series were carried out using Pearson's chi-square test, and in the event of non-validity of this test and comparison of 2 percentages, using Fisher's two-tailed exact test.

3. **Search for factors contributing to poor asthma control :**

The search for risk factors was carried out by calculating the Odds Ratio (OR), which represents the number of times by which the risk of an event is multiplied in the event of exposure to a factor compared with non-exposure. In order to identify the risk factors independently linked to the event, we conducted a multivariate analysis using logistic regression.Multivariate analysis was used to calculate adjusted ORs, measuring the specific role of each factor. In all statistical tests, the significance level (p) was set at 0.05. The alpha risk of error was set at 5%.

VI. Collection of bibliographical data :

We used the Science Direct and Pub Med websites to search for articles using the following keywords: asthma, adolescent and control.

VII. Ethical considerations and conflicts of interest :

We have no conflicts of interest in relation to this study.

RESULTS

A. Characteristics of the study population :

Based on GINA 2018, two groups were identified: a controlled group and an uncontrolled group.

I. Characteristics of the controlled group :

This group included 28 adolescents with asthma.

1. Epidemiological characteristics :

The mean age was 13 years, with extremes of 10 and 18 years. Males predominated, with a sex ratio of 1.8.
Thirteen adolescents (46.4%) were exposed to passive smoking and n o n e of them were active smokers.

Socioeconomic conditions were good to average in 92.9% of cases (26).

Humidity was present in the homes of 9 adolescents (32.1%).

A pet was present in the patient's environment in 28.6% of cases (8).

Three teenagers were obese, as shown in Figure 1.

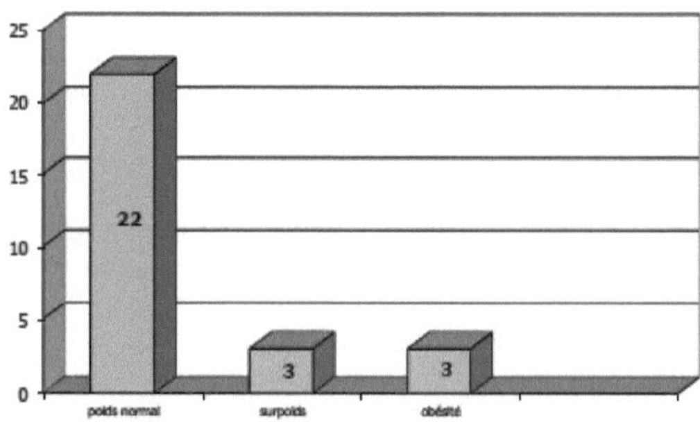

Figure 1: Distribution of patients according to weight (controlled group).

2. Clinical features :

a. Age at onset and diagnosis of asthma :

The average age at onset of the disease was 5 years, with extremes of 1 and 11 years. Asthma began in adolescence in 4 patients.

The average duration of the disease was 7.9 years (1-15).

The average age at diagnosis was 6.5 years. Delayed diagnosis was noted in 12 cases (42.9%).
Table I shows the phenotypes of the disease as a function of age of onset.

Table I: Asthma phenotypes according to age of onset (controlled group).

Phenotypes	Persistent whistlers early onset (<3 years)	Persistent whistlers late onset (>3 years)	Whistlers late (>6 years)	Total
N	12	8	8	28
%	42,8%	28,6%	28,6%	100%

b. Allergic nature :

Skin tests were carried out on 21 adolescents in the control group. They were positive in 11 cases (52.4%).Mites were implicated in all cases. Sensitisation to Blomia Tropicalis was also noted in one case.

c. Associated atopic symptoms :

Allergic rhinitis was present in 13 adolescents (46.4%). It was associated with allergic asthma in 66.7% of cases (6 out of 9 cases).Allergic conjunctivitis was present in one adolescent (3.6%). Family atopy was found in 17 adolescents (60.7%).Sixteen adolescents (57.1%) had a family history of asthma.The combination of family and personal atopy concerned nine adolescents (32.1%).

d. Characteristics of asthma :

* The severity of the disease :

Asthma was persistent in 92.9% of cases (26).

Table II shows the severity of asthma in our 28 controlled asthmatic adolescents.

Table II: Disease severity (controlled group).

Severity of the disease	N	%
Mild asthma	20	71,4
Moderate asthma	8	28,6
Severe asthma	0	0
Total	28	100

* Disease profile over the last 12 months :

- Exacerbations: one patient has had a moderate exacerbation in the last 12 months.

- Hospital admissions: one patient was hospitalised for a moderate asthma attack.

- School attendance and sporting activity: no asthma-related difficulties at school or restrictions on sporting activity were recorded in the controlled group.

3. Psychological assessment :

It involved six adolescents (21.4%) and abnormalities were noted in three cases. In one case, the teenager showed anxiety.In the second case, maternal anxiety and depression were observed.In the third case, there was depression in the child and anxiety and depression in the mother. In addition, one mother was found to have misconceptions about background treatment, with the result that she refused to give the treatment.

4. Respiratory function :

a. Peak expiratory flow (PEF):

It was measured in 25 patients. It was normal in 88% of cases. In the other cases, it was moderately reduced.

The results of the EPD values as a function of the theoretical value are summarised in Table III.

Table III: PEF values as a function of the theoretical value (controlled group).

DEP	N	%
> 80% theoretical	22	88
60-80% theoretical	3	12
< 60% theoretical	0	0
Total	25	100

b. Functional respiratory examination (FRE) :

All patients in this group were investigated by spirometry. Mean FEV1 was 2.2 litres. Normal FEV1 was found in 42.9% of cases (12).The average Tiffeneau index was 83.4%. An obstructive syndrome was present in 60.7% of adolescents in the control group (17 cases). The results are summarised in Figure 2.

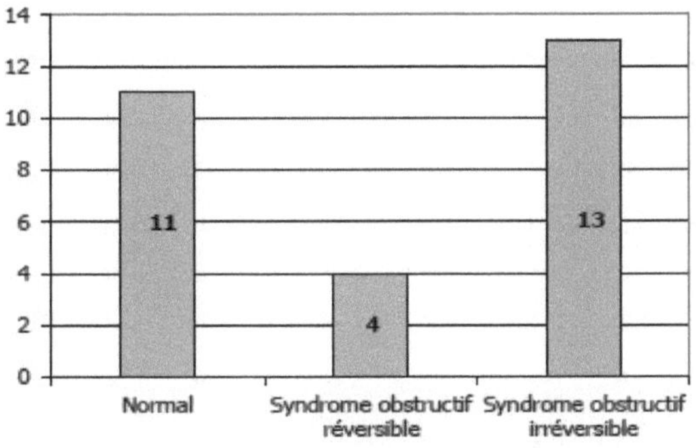

Figure 2: Spirometry results (controlled group).

5. Biological investigations :

* Eosinophilic polymorphonuclear cells: these were found in 24 patients. Hypereosinophilia was found in 54.2% of cases (13).

* Total IgE: this was measured in 4 patients. They were increased in all cases.

6. Therapeutic characteristics :

a. Background treatment :

* **Inhaled corticosteroids:** only two patients in this group were not taking inhaled corticosteroids.

Inhaled corticosteroid therapy was the background treatment used alone in 67.9% of cases (19/26).The doses of inhaled corticosteroids were low in 61.5% of cases, medium in 30.8% and high in 7.7%.

* **Long-acting beta-2** mimetics: used in 7 patients in combination with inhaled corticosteroids (25%).

b. Type of inhalation system :

The metered dose inhaler was the most commonly used inhalation system (71.4%). The metered dose inhaler combined with the inhalation chamber was used in 14.3% of cases. The different inhalation techniques are summarised in Figure 3.

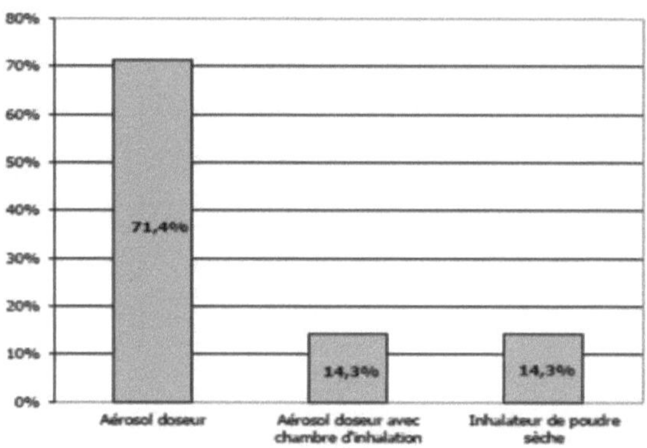

Figure 3: Répartition selon le type du système d'inhalation
(groupe contrôlé).

Figure 3: Distribution by type of inhalation system (controlled group).

c. Inhalation technique :

It was evaluated in 23 patients. It was good in all cases.

d. Therapeutic compliance :

It was judged to be good in 75% of patients (21).

II. Characteristics of the uncontrolled group :

This group included 22 adolescents with asthma (44%).

1. Epidemiological characteristics :

The mean age was 12.7 years, with extremes of 10 and 16 years. Males predominated, with a sex ratio of 1.8. Half of the adolescents (11) were exposed to passive smoking and none of them were active smokers.Socio-economic conditions were poor in 13.7% of cases (3). Dampness was present in the homes of 14 adolescents (63.6%). A pet was present in the patient's environment in 18.2% of cases (4). Two adolescents were overweight and none were obese (weight assessed in 21 adolescents in this group) (Figure 4).

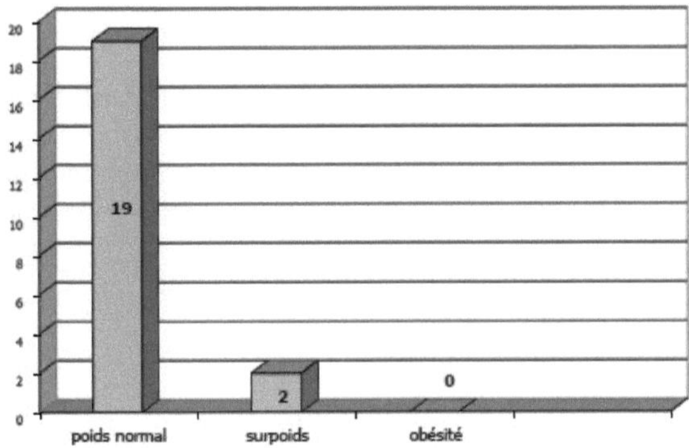

Figure 4: Distribution of patients according to weight (uncontrolled group).

2. Clinical features :

a. Age at onset and diagnosis of asthma :

The average age at onset of the disease was 4 years, with extremes of 1 and 12 years. Asthma began in adolescence in 3 patients.The average duration of the disease was 8.7 years (1-14).The average age at diagnosis was 5.7 years. Delayed diagnosis was noted in 13 cases (59.1%).

Table IV shows the phenotypes of the disease as a function of age of onset.

Table IV: Asthma phenotypes according to age of onset (uncontrolled group).

Phenotypes	Persistent whistlers	Persistent whistlers	Whistlers	Total
	early onset	late onset	late (>6 years)	
	(<3 years)	(>3 years)		
N	13	4	5	22
%	59,1%	18,2%	22,7%	100%

b. Allergic nature :

Skin tests were carried out on 17 adolescents in the uncontrolled group. They were positive in 10 cases (58.8%).House dust mites were the allergens most frequently implicated (8 cases). They were associated with Blomia Tropicalis in two cases and moulds in one case. The other two cases involved sensitisation to grasses and a combination of grasses and cereals respectively.

c. Associated atopic symptoms :

Allergic rhinitis was present in 8 adolescents (36.4%). It was associated with allergic asthma in 75% of cases (6 out of 8 cases).Allergic conjunctivitis was present in 3 adolescents (13.6%). Familial atopy was found in 13 adolescents (59.1%). Seven adolescents (31.8%) had a family history of asthma. The combination of family and personal atopy concerned 6 adolescents (27.3%).

d. Characteristics of asthma :

* Severity of asthma :

Asthma was persistent in all cases.

Table V shows the severity of asthma in our 22 uncontrolled asthmatic adolescents.

Table V: Disease severity (uncontrolled group).

Severity of the disease	N	%
Mild asthma	14	63,6
Moderate asthma	8	36,4
Severe asthma	0	0
Total	22	100

* Disease profile over the last 12 months :

- Exacerbations: Four patients had at least one exacerbation in the previous 12 months. Exacerbations were frequent in two cases.

- Hospital admissions: one patient was admitted to intensive care for a severe asthma attack.

- Schooling: seven adolescents (31.8%) experienced difficulties at school, including two who dropped out.

- Sports activity: limited in 6 adolescents (27.3%) because of their asthma.

3. Psychological assessment :

Eight adolescents (36.4%) were involved. An abnormality was noted in one case. One adolescent was depressed.The interview with the psychologist also revealed some of the parents' misconceptions about asthma. These included misconceptions about the adverse effects of disease-modifying therapy, resulting in the refusal to give the treatment to the teenager.

4. Respiratory function :

a. Peak expiratory flow :

It was measured in 21 adolescents. It was significantly reduced in 14.3% of cases and moderately reduced in 33.3%.The results of the EPD values as a function of the theoretical value are summarised in Table VI.

Table VI: PEF values as a function of the theoretical value (uncontrolled group).

DEP	N	%
> 80% theoretical	11	52,4
60-80% theoretical	7	33,3
< 60% theoretical	3	14,3
Total	21	100

b. Respiratory function test :

Twenty adolescents in this group were investigated by spirometry. The mean FEV1 was 2.2 litres. Normal FEV1 was found in 55% of cases (11). The average Tiffeneau index was 84.3%.An obstructive syndrome was present in 13 adolescents (65%). The spirometry results are summarised in figure 5.

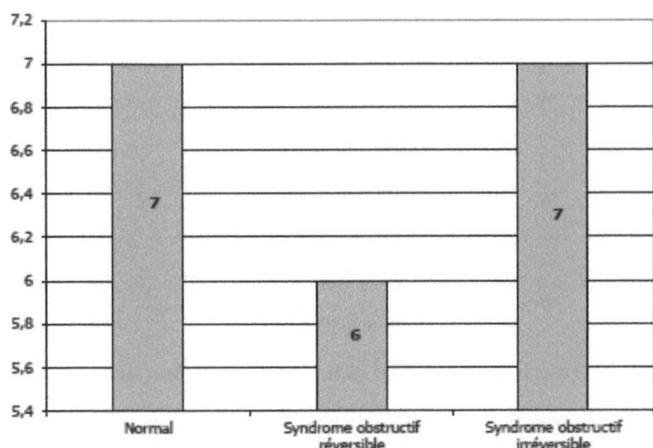

Figure 5: Spirometry results (uncontrolled group).

5. Biological investigations :

* Eosinophilic polymorphs :

They were detected in 21 patients. Hypereosinophilia was found in 47.6% of cases (10).

* Total IgE :

They were measured in 6 patients. They were increased in all cases.

6. Therapeutic characteristics :

a. Background treatment :

* **Inhaled corticosteroid therapy :**

It was the background treatment used alone in most cases (68.2%).

The doses of inhaled corticosteroidswerelowin 68.2% of cases, medium in 9.1% and high in 22.7%.

* **Long-acting beta-2 mimetics :**

They were used in 7 patients (31.8%) in combination with inhaled corticosteroids.

b. Type of inhalation system :

The metered dose inhaler was the most commonly used inhalation system (68.2%). The metered dose inhaler and inhalation chamber were used in 9.1% of cases. The different inhalation techniques are summarised in Figure 6.

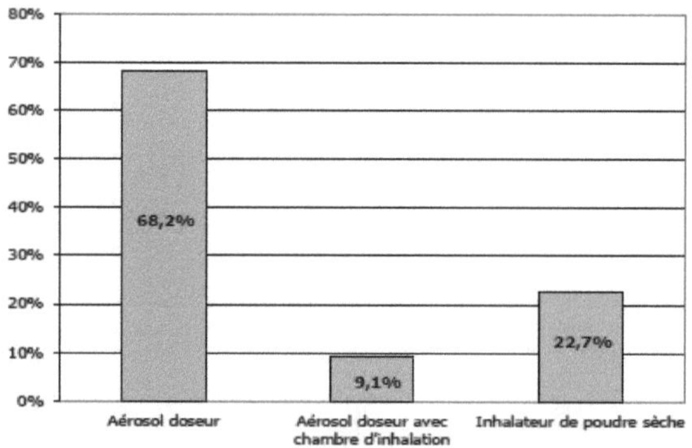

Figure 6: Distribution by type of inhalation system (uncontrolled group).

c. Inhalation technique :

It was assessed in 12 patients. It was poor in 16.7% of cases (2).

d. Therapeutic compliance :

It was judged to be poor in half the cases (11).

B. Factors influencing asthma control :

1. Age :

No statistically significant relationship was found between mean age at assessment and level of asthma control (p=0.67).Similarly, there was no significant relationship between early age of onset (before the age of 6) and level of asthma control in adolescence (p=0.64).

2. Genre :

There was no statistically significant relationship between gender and asthma control (p=0.96) (Table VII).

Table VII: Gender and asthma control.

	Controlled	Not controlled	P
Male	18 (56,3%)	14 (43,7%)	
Female	10 (55,6%)	8 (44,4%)	0,96

3. Obesity :

Overweight did not significantly affect asthma control (p=0.43) (table VIII).

Table VIII: Distribution of adolescents according to weight.

	Controlled	Not controlled	P
Obesity/overweight	6 (75%)	2 (25%)	
Normal weight	22 (53,7%)	19 (46,3%)	0,43

4. Passive smoking :

No statistically significant relationship was found between exposure to passive smoking and the level of asthma control in adolescents (p=0.8) (table IX).

Table IX: Distribution of adolescents according to exposure to passive smoking.

	Controlled	Not controlled	P
Tobacco (+)	13 (54,2%)	11 (45,8%)	
Tobacco (-)	15 (57,7%)	11 (42,3%)	0,8

5. Humidity in the home :

The presence of a high level of humidity in the home was significantly correlated with poor asthma control (p=0.027) (table X).

Table X: Distribution of adolescents according to humidity in the home.

	Controlled	Not controlled	P
Humidity (+)	9 (39,1%)	14 (60,9%)	
Humidity (-)	19 (70,4%)	8 (29,6%)	0,027

6. Contact with pets :

The presence of pets in the environment of asthmatic adolescents was more frequent in the controlled group (28.6%) than in the uncontrolled group (18.2%). The difference was not statistically significant (p=0.39).

7. Socio-economic conditions (CSE) :

ESCs were worse in the uncontrolled group, but there was no significant association with asthma control (p=0.64) (table XI).

Table XI: Breakdown of adolescents by SSC.

	Controlled	Not controlled	P
Good/average	26 (57,8%)	19 (42,2%)	
Bad	2 (40%)	3 (60%)	0,64

8. Duration of disease :

The mean duration of the disease in the whole group was 8.3 years ± 4.3 (1-15). Adolescents with controlled asthma had a shorter average disease duration (7.9 years ± 4.1) than those with uncontrolled asthma (8.7 years ± 1), but the difference was not significant (p=0.5).

9. Severity of asthma :

There was no statistically significant correlation between asthma severity and asthma control (p=0.36), although in this series the adolescents all had mild to moderate asthma (table XII).

Table XII: Distribution of adolescents according to asthma severity.

	Controlled	Not controlled	P
Mild asthma	20 (58,8%)	14 (41,2%)	
Moderate asthma	8 (50%)	8 (50%)	0,36

10. Respiratory function :

a. Peak expiratory flow :

A decrease in PEF below the threshold of 80% of the theoretical value for height was significantly correlated with the level of asthma control (p=0.018) (table XIII).

Table XIII: Breakdown of adolescents by DEP.

	Controlled	Not controlled	P
PEF > 80% theoretical	22 (58,8%)	12 (41,2%)	
DEP :!:' 80% theoretical	3 (25%)	9 (75%)	0,018

b. Respiratory function test :

No statistically significant relationship was found between the presence of an intercritical obstructive syndrome and the level of asthma control (p=0.76) (table XIV).

Table XIV: Distribution of adolescents according to intercritical LFT.

	Controlled	Not controlled	P
Pathological EFR	17 (56,7%)	13 (43,3%)	
EFR normal	11 (61,1%)	7 (38,9%)	0,76

11. Atopic skin :

a. Familial atopy :

There was no statistically significant relationship between the presence of family atopy and the level of asthma control in adolescence (p=0.52), including for a family history of asthma (p=0.07).

b. Personal atopy :

*** Allergic rhinitis (AR):**

Of the 50 adolescents included in this study, 22 had associated allergic rhinitis. Eight had uncontrolled asthma.There was no statistically significant relationship between the presence of allergic rhinitis and the level of asthma control (p=0.335) (table XV).

Table XV: Allergic rhinitis and level of asthma control.

	Controlled	Not controlled	P
Allergic rhinitis (+)	14 (63,6%)	8 (36,4%)	
Allergic rhinitis (-)	14 (50%)	14 (50%)	0,335

*** Allergic conjunctivitis (AC) :**

It was more frequent in the uncontrolled group (13.6%) than in the controlled group (3.6%), but the difference was not significant (p=0.3).

*** Hypereosinophilia :**

The frequency of hypereosinophilia in the controlled group (54.2%) and in the uncontrolled group (47.6%) was comparable, and the difference was not statistically significant (p=0.66).

12. Skin sensitisation :

Of the 38 adolescents who were prick-tested for pneumallergens, 21 had positive skin tests. Ten of these (47.6%) were uncontrolled. There was no statistically significant relationship between skin test positivity and level of asthma control (p=0.69) (table XVI).

Table XVI: Skin sensitisation and level of asthma control.

	Controlled	Not controlled	P
Skin tests (+)	11 (52,4%)	10 (47,6%)	
Skin tests (-)	10 (58,8%)	7 (41,2%)	0,69

13. Background treatment :

Treatment was initiated in all the asthmatic adolescents included in our study except two patients in the control group. Treatment consisted of either inhaled corticosteroids (ICS) alone or a combination of ICS and long-acting beta-2 mimetics (LABMs). There was no statistically significant relationship between the type of background treatment and asthma control (p=0.71) (table XVII).

Table XVII: Background treatment and asthma control.

	Controlled	Not controlled	P
CSI	19 (55,9%)	15 (44,1%)	
CSI + BLDA	7 (50%)	7 (50%)	0,71

14. Use of the inhalation chamber (IC) :

IC was used more frequently in the controlled group (80%) than in the uncontrolled group (20%). However, there was no correlation with the level of asthma control (p=0.36) (table XVIII).

Table XVIII: Inhalation chamber use and asthma control.

	Controlled	Not controlled	P
CI (+)	4 (80%)	1 (20%)	
CI (-)	24 (53,3%)	21 (46,7%)	0,36

15. Inhalation technique :

It was assessed in only 12 adolescents in the uncontrolled group (54.6%). No statistically significant relationship was found between the quality of inhalation technique and the level of asthma control (p=0.11) (table XIX).

Table XIX: Inhalation technique and asthma control.

Inhalation technique	Controlled	Not controlled	P
Good	23 (69,7%)	10 (30,3%)	
Wrong	0 (0%)	2 (100%)	0,11

16. Therapeutic compliance :

A statistically significant relationship was found between poor compliance and poor asthma control in adolescents (p=0.002) (table XX).

Table XX: Therapeutic compliance and asthma control.

	Controlled	Not controlled	P
Good compliance	21 (75%)	7 (25%)	
Poor compliance	7 (31,8%)	15 (68,2%)	0,002

C. Effects of asthma :

1. School :

All patients with well-controlled asthma did not experience problems at school. There was a statistically significant relationship between poor asthma control and educational delay in adolescents (p=0.002) (table XXI).

Table XXI: Impact of asthma on adolescents' schooling.

	Controlled	Not controlled	P
School delay	0 (0%)	7 (100%)	
Normal schooling	28 (65,1%)	15 (34,9%)	0,002

2. Sports activity :

All adolescents in the control group had normal sporting activity. A significant correlation was found between poor asthma control and limitation of sporting activity (p=0.005) (table XXII).

Table XXII: Impact of asthma on sporting activity in adolescents.

Sports activities	Controlled	Not controlled	P
Limited	0 (0%)	6 (100%)	
Normal	28 (63,6%)	16 (36,4%)	0,005

D. Multivariate study :

Only poor compliance was correlated with poor asthma control in adolescents (**p=0.011; OR=6.42 [1.86-22.2]**).

DISCUSSION

Achieving and maintaining asthma control has become the goal of international guidelines, and assessment of asthma control has become the mainstay of asthma management [7]. Adolescence is a period of transition characterised by denial of asthma, non-compliance with treatment and poor control of the disease.To determine the factors influencing asthma control in adolescents, we conducted a cross-sectional study with retrospective data collection and comparison of two groups of adolescents with asthma: a controlled group of 28 patients and an uncontrolled group of 22 patients.Asthma control was judged according to GINA 2018 [7]. The poor control factors identified in our study were: a high level of humidity in the home, a reduced intercritical peak expiratory flow and poor compliance with treatment. Nevertheless, our work has certain limitations:

*Type of study :

A case-control study would be more powerful than a cross-sectional study with random selection of cases from among all asthma patients (the cases would be uncontrolled adolescents).

*Information bias :

Given the retrospective nature of the study, data collection was confronted with a number of data gaps.

*Selection bias :

The study took place in a referral paediatric respirology department. Asthma patients referred to this department generally have severe asthma or asthma that is difficult to control.

A. Epidemiological characteristics :

I. Age :

The hypothesis that the prognosis of childhood asthma differs depending on whether the age of onset is before 3 years or later (between 3 and 6 years) was first described in the classification of the Tucson Respiratory Study.[10]. Children suffering from recurrent wheezing with a late onset are more likely to be more likely to have asthma that persists throughout childhood, adolescence and sometimes adulthood than those with early-onset recurrent wheezing, which is often transient over the course of a lifetime. Bouzigon et al [11] have confirmed a genetic basis for the age of onset of asthma. Polymorphisms in genes located on chromosome 17q21 (such as the gene coding for ORMDL3) are associated with an early-onset asthma phenotype triggered by respiratory infections, with a more favourable prognosis (remission of symptoms in adulthood).Asthma with onset before the age of 12 or with late onset after the age of 12 can also be defined. Onset before the age of 12 is more often associated with atopy, whereas asthma after the age of 12 is more associated with females, bronchial obstruction and active smoking [12]. In our study, asthma started at pre-school age in 13 patients (26%). We found no statistically significant association between early age of onset (before age 6) and asthma control in adolescence (p=0.64).

II. Genre :

After puberty, asthma becomes more frequent and more severe in girls, especially in the case of early puberty, suggesting a role for sex hormones in the genesis of asthma. The age at which this change occurs varies according to studies, from 11 to 18 years [13]. Puberty is marked by changes in circulating levels of sex hormones. In boys, higher levels of androgens are associated with better lung function, whereas in girls, higher levels of circulating oestrogens may have small but significant deleterious effects on lung function [14].A study carried out in Boston showed that hospitalisation for asthma attacks was more frequent in boys before the age of 14 and significantly more frequent in girls from adolescence onwards [15]. This was confirmed by Varraso, who found that young girls who had undergone early puberty and were obese were at risk of severe asthma. This is explained by hormonal changes [16].Sears [17] reported that female gender is a factor in the persistence of asthma in adolescence. In our series, males predominated (64%) with a sex ratio of 1.8. There was no significant relationship between gender and level of asthma control (p=0.96).

III. Passive smoking :

Passive smoking is a major public health problem. In the AIRMAG survey [18], which studied the prevalence and management of paediatric asthma in the Maghreb countries, passive smoking reached 31.9% in Morocco, 41.6% in Algeria and 53.3% in Tunisia. In a cross-sectional study of 3187 children aged 8 to 13 from eight Portuguese cities, 32.6% were exposed to passive smoking in the home [19].A secondary cross-sectional analysis of the PATH (Population Assessment of Tobacco and Health) study conducted in the United States, which included 2187 non-smoking asthmatic adolescents aged 12 to 17, found a passive smoking rate of 28.9% [20]. In this study, exposure to passive smoking for more than one hour in the last seven days was associated with more respiratory problems, less physical activity and sleep disturbance. In addition, there was a greater risk of asthma attacks and of seeking urgent care.Exposure to passive smoking, even at low levels, is associated with an increased risk of poorly controlled asthma and asthma exacerbation, with a dose-response relationship [21]. De Blic [22] also found that passive smoking significantly affects asthma control in children (P<0.001). In fact, only 20% of patients exposed to passive smoking had well-controlled asthma.Passive smoking worsens the severity of asthma by affecting the balance between Treg and Th17 lymphocytes. FoxP3 and TGF-□ levels decrease, while serum IL17-A and IL-23 levels increase as asthma progresses [23]. Passive smoking also interferes with the background treatment of asthma by reducing the response to ICS treatment. In a study carried out by Alterman et al [24], comparing supervised ICS treatment in a school setting with treatment instituted in the usual setting, in 180 children aged 3 to 7 years, it was found that showed that the improvement observed in the first group was only significant in children who were not exposed to passive smoking. Smoking cessation reduces the frequency of asthma symptoms, improves lung function and restores response to corticosteroids [25]. In our study, approximately half of the adolescents, in both the controlled and uncontrolled groups, were exposed to passive smoking. There was no statistically significant association between passive smoking and asthma control in adolescence (p=0.8).

IV. Obesity :

Overweight and obesity are the cause of cardiovascular, metabolic, respiratory and orthopaedic complications.... In paediatrics, respiratory complications are the most frequent. The incidences of obesity and asthma follow a parallel progression [26]. In a study of 7,505 children aged between 4 and 17 years, Von Mutius et al [27] showed that BMI was an independent risk factor for the development of asthma. They concluded that an appropriate weight reduction strategy in children could help to reduce the incidence of asthma in childhood. Similarly, Castro-Rodriguez et al established from the Tucson cohort that becoming obese between the ages of 6 and 11 in girls increased the risk of developing asthma by a factor of 7 at the age of 13 [28].Asthma is an inflammatory disease of the bronchi and obesity is considered to be a pro-inflammatory condition. Based on fat biopsies taken from 18 obese adolescents and compared with those taken from five control children, Sbarbati et al showed signs of chronic inflammation in obese patients: degeneration of adipocytes, inflammatory cellular infiltrates, microgranulomatous lesions and fibrosis [29]. Shore reported that adipocytes could secrete numerous mediators and cytokines involved in the inflammatory response, particularly in the bronchial system [30].The role of adipokines, and in particular leptin, in obese asthma is debated. Leptin secretion is increased in the obese and has a pro-inflammatory effect. Treatment of sensitised mice with leptin increased allergen-induced bronchial hyperreactivity but did not affect airway influx. of eosinophils or TH2 cytokine expression, suggesting that leptin is capable of increasing bronchial hyperresponsiveness by a mechanism independent of TH2 inflammation [30,31]. Unlike leptin, adiponectin, another hormone secreted by adipose tissue, has an anti-inflammatory action by inhibiting the synthesis of certain cytokines such as TNF (tumour necrosis factor) alpha or IL6, and by promoting the synthesis of anti-inflammatory molecules such as IL10. The consequences of obesity on respiratory function have also been clarified [32]. There is an increase in oxygen consumption at rest, minute ventilation and ventilatory work.In a study of the influence of childhood growth on asthma and lung function, Sonnenschein-van der voort et al showed that weight gain during the first three months of life was associated with asthma and bronchial hyperresponsiveness at the ages of 8 and 17 [33]. These various studies underline the importance of identifying obesity early, from the very first months of life, and ensuring that it is properly managed.In our study, eight adolescents (16.3%) were overweight. There was no statistically significant relationship between overweight and asthma control (p=0.43).

V. Humidity in the home :

High levels of humidity in the home encourage the growth of moulds and bacteria, with moulds emitting bioaerosols and spores as well as volatile compounds [34].In a study of asthma patients aged 5 to 44 and a control group, Williamson et al [35] found that asthma severity was significantly correlated with humidity levels and mould growth in the home, with a dose-response relationship. In another study involving 106 patients with allergic rhinitis or allergic rhinitis with asthma, humidity was a factor that aggravated symptoms in allergic asthmatics, but there was no significant relationship with asthma severity [34].
Nicolai et al [36], in a study involving 155 adolescents (mean age = 13.5 years), found that risk factors for persistence of hyperresponsiveness bronchial hyperreactivity during childhood,

symptoms triggered by allergen exposure and dampness in the home. Action to reduce humidity in the home may therefore have a positive impact on asthma-related morbidity [35]. In our study, the presence of dampness in the home was positively correlated with poor asthma control (p=0.027).

VI. Contact with pets :

Epidemiological studies of the relationship between exposure to pet allergens and asthma exacerbation have produced conflicting results. However, there is evidence to support this relationship. The results of the meta-analysis by Apelberg et al [37] showed that exposure to a pet was associated with an increased risk of sibilance in children aged 6 and over, whereas no association was observed in younger children. The case-control study by Strachan et al [38] showed that the presence of pets in the home was an independent risk factor for severe episodes of sibilance in adolescents aged 11 to 16.The retrospective study by Sarpong et al [39] of young asthmatics aged between 5 and 18 also identified the presence of a cat in the home as a risk factor for hospitalisation for asthma. Animal avoidance is recommended in the management of patients with allergic asthma in order to reduce airway inflammation, with the corollary of reducing bronchial hyperresponsiveness and improving lung function [40].In our study, the presence of pets in the environment of asthmatic adolescents was reported in twelve cases (24%). It was not significantly related to the level of asthma control (p=0.39).

VII. Socio-economic conditions :

Among social factors, low socio-economic status has one of the strongest and most consistent associations with the morbidity and mortality of several diseases, including childhood asthma [41,42]. Children from low socio-economic backgrounds are much more likely to be hospitalised or to visit emergency departments for asthma. They also have more severe symptoms and exacerbations than children with asthma from higher socio-economic backgrounds [43,44]. In children with asthma, low socio-economic status is associated with a tendency to express inflammatory profiles, including higher levels of eosinophils and greater TH2 cytokine responses [45,46]. This relationship between low socio-economic status and these immune processes is largely explained by chronic stress and threat perception [46]. This suggests that stress disrupts immune processes in children with asthma, which may shift responses towards a TH2 profile and sensitise the TH2 system to a more aggressive response after allergen exposure [47,48,49]. In addition, chronic stress can affect other biological systems such as the hypothalamic-pituitary-adrenal axis, which becomes less active [50].People with low socio-economic status are more likely to live in areas with high levels of exposure to air pollution, and to live in substandard housing [51], which increases exposure to cockroach and mould antigens [52].The "Moving to Opportunity" study, carried out in Boston in the United States, enabled families from areas of extreme poverty living in social housing to move to flats in better neighbourhoods. The families who moved felt that their children's asthma was less severe after the move [53]. In a study involving 150 asthmatic children aged 9 to 17, Chen et al [54] found that a higher level of parental education was associated with better control of the home environment and lower exposure to tobacco.But the effects of socio-economic status on asthma are transmitted by mechanisms that are not limited to environmental exposures. Households on the lowest incomes are more likely to bear a heavy financial burden in managing their children's asthma, have a higher rate of recourse to emergency care and experience more school absenteeism. due to asthma [55].Children were less likely to receive ICS if they came from low-income families [56,57]. In a literature review of articles published between 1997 and 2016 on adherence in paediatric asthma (0-25 years), Gray et al [58] found that socioeconomic status was one of the most important factors correlated with adherence to inhaled corticosteroid therapy. Young people from low socio-economic backgrounds were at high risk of non-adherence. In our study, there was no significant relationship between socio-economic status and asthma control (p=0.64). Nevertheless, financial problems were noted in the families of five adolescents in the uncontrolled group; these were the cause of discontinuation of treatment in two cases, and of poor compliance in the other three. On the other hand, parents' low level of education and misconceptions about asthma were at the root of poor compliance in five cases.

B. Clinical features :

I. Age of illness :

In our study, adolescents with controlled asthma had a shorter disease duration (7.9 years) than those with uncontrolled asthma (8.7 years), with a non-significant difference (p=0.5). In a clinical trial conducted in children aged between 7 and 16 years, Jonasson et al [59] found that compliance with treatment decreased over time, which may explain the influence of the duration of the disease on asthma control. The decrease in compliance was proportional to the duration of treatment; it fell from 77% at 3 months to 27% at 27 months of treatment. The length of time asthma has been present can theoretically influence disease control. Persistent asthma is associated with changes in the bronchial walls, as part of bronchial remodelling. These abnormalities are reflected in the progressive development of residual bronchial obstruction, which may or may not be sensitive to bronchodilators or even inhaled corticosteroids. Bronchial remodelling could be a parallel phenomenon to airway inflammation and not a consequence of it. systematically secondary to it [60].

II. Disease severity :

The severity of asthma takes into account the history of the disease over a sufficiently long period, usually 6 to 12 months [4].In a prospective study of 220 adolescents with persistent asthma, Vidal et al [61] found that asthma control according to the ACT test decreased with increasing disease severity (p=0.001). Between the ages of 6 and 12, exposure to allergens and exertion appear to be the factors most responsible for inducing exacerbations [62]. In younger children, viral respiratory infections appear to be the most frequent cause [63,64]. Severe asthma is more common in adolescence, and psychosocial factors are increasingly associated with the severity of the disease at this age [65,66]. Control and severity of the disease are two independent concepts; severe asthma can be controlled and moderate asthma uncontrolled [67]. Asthma control must be achieved whatever the severity of the asthma. In our series, no severe form of asthma was observed. Asthma was mild in 66% of cases and moderate in 34%. Exacerbations were more frequent in the uncontrolled group (4 cases) than in the controlled group (1 case).There was no statistically significant relationship between severity and asthma control (p=0.36).

III. Associated atopic symptoms :

The atopic symptoms associated with asthma in our study were rhinitis and allergic conjunctivitis.

a. Rhinitis :

Rhinitis is more common in asthmatic children [68,69]. Unlike in adults, the development of asthma in children with rhinitis is often associated with allergy [70]. Several studies, both in adults [71,72] and children [68,69,73], report the aggravating role of rhinitis in the severity of asthma and its poor control.Other studies mention the beneficial role of rhinitis treatment in asthmatic patients. In a prospective study of adolescent and adult patients, Crystal-Peters et al [74] found that local treatment of rhinitis significantly reduced asthma attacks, night-time awakenings and absenteeism due to asthma. Similarly, Yu et al [75] showed in a retrospective study of asthmatic children aged between 2 and 18 years that treatment with nasal corticosteroids and/or 2ème generation antihistamines significantly reduced the incidence of asthma exacerbations in the group with allergic rhinitis. In our study, 44% of adolescents had rhinitis. We found no significant relationship between the presence of rhinitis and asthma control (p=0.34).

b. Allergic conjunctivitis :

In our study, allergic conjunctivitis affected 13.6% of patients in the uncontrolled group. There was no significant association with asthma control.

IV. Allergic nature of asthma :

There is a strong relationship between allergen sensitisation and asthma [76]. The type of sensitisation varies according to the population studied.Although allergy is strongly associated with childhood asthma, the question of the association between the intensity of allergenic sensitisation and the severity and/or control of asthma is controversial [77].

In a study of 400 asthmatic children aged 7 to 18, Carrol et al [78] found a significant relationship between atopy markers (IgE, skin tests) and asthma severity.Another study of 24 children followed up until the age of 11 showed that the risk of developing severe, uncontrolled asthma was higher in children in whom allergen sensitisation had been detected before the age of six [79]. Sears et al [17], in a cohort of children followed prospectively from the age of 9 to 26, found that allergy is one of the risk factors for the transition from childhood asthma to adulthood.In contrast, the EGEA study of asthmatic children found no link between atopy markers (IgE, blood eosinophils, skin tests) and disease severity [80]. In our study, 55.3% of adolescents had positive skin tests, but there was no correlation with asthma control (p=0.69).

C. Psychological factor :

Anxiety and depressive disorders are more common in adolescents with asthma than in their healthy peers. These psychopathological difficulties are observed especially in cases of severe asthma.A meta-analysis reports a 27% prevalence of depression among adolescents with asthma, which is more than double that of adolescents without asthma [81].

Bender [82] has put forward a number of hypotheses explaining the relationship between asthma and depressive symptoms. On the one hand, poor asthma control may cause distress leading to depressive symptoms. On the other hand, depression can cause poor adherence to treatment or an increase in chronic inflammation leading to functional and physical dysfunction. Finally, some individuals may have a genetic predisposition that underlies both asthma severity and depressive symptoms. With regard to anxiety disorders, in a meta-analysis of 7000 asthmatic children and adolescents, the prevalence of anxiety disorders was 22.7%, which is three times the prevalence reported in healthy individuals [83]. A particular feature of asthmatic adolescents is the higher frequency of social anxiety. This is probably due to the fear of negative reactions from peers and increasing embarrassment in social situations [84].Some adolescents with asthma are at greater risk of developing anxiety disorders. The risk factors identified by various studies are: being Caucasian, female, being a smoker, living in a single-parent family, newly diagnosed asthma, severe asthma and the presence of family problems [84,85]. Symptoms of anxiety (shortness of breath, rapid heart rate) and depressive disorders (insomnia, fatigue) may overlap with asthma symptoms [85], making their diagnosis sometimes difficult.Furthermore, teenagers are often exposed to highly stressful situations and are at greater risk of developing chronic stress. Anxiety disorders may be one of the markers or a consequence of this chronic stress. Chronic stress can have a direct effect on asthma by creating a pro-inflammatory climate through down-regulation of glucocorticoid and catecholamine receptors, and by reducing the response to certain treatments such as short-acting bronchodilators [86,87,88]. Similarly, high levels of chronic family stress in young asthmatics stimulate the production in vitro of cytokines involved in asthma, including interleukin (IL)-5 and IL-13, and mobilise and activate eosinophils in vivo [89].

Stress may also have an effect on asthma through indirect mechanisms, including smoking, overweight or obesity and reduced adherence to treatment [86,90,91]. Several studies have established a link between perceived stress and asthma symptoms in adolescents. In a prospective study involving 20 low-income asthmatic adolescents, stressful situations (arguments, disagreements with parents, etc.) were associated with worsening of asthma symptoms in the hours following the stressful events [92]. Similar findings were reported in a study of 61 adolescents aged 10 to 20 years (38 of whom had asthma), which revealed that the fraction of exhaled nitric oxide increased approximately 45 min after acute stress (family conflict), but only in children with asthma and low socio-economic status [93]. These various studies highlight the fact that repeated stressful situations can exacerbate airway inflammation and trigger asthma symptoms.Anxiety and depressive disorders aggravate asthma-related morbidity in adolescents. In a randomised controlled trial involving 277 asthmatic adolescents aged 12 to 16 years, Shankar et al [94] found that the group with depressive symptoms (28%) had more severe asthma and more frequent use of acute care (p<0.001). Similarly, adolescents with with depression reported lower asthma-related quality of life (p<0.001), less sleep (p<0.001) and greater limitation of physical activity.In another study, Bender [82] found that the presence of anxiety and/or depression in adolescents with asthma was associated with poor asthma control, increased use of healthcare, reduced quality of life, poor adherence to treatment and poor therapeutic outcome. Furthermore, a dysfunctional emotional climate in the family can trigger asthma symptoms and affect the severity of the disease [95,96]. In a study by Wolf et al [97], stress and depression, initially identified in the parents, increased the inflammatory profile of the children over a 6-month period. This was observed in both healthy and asthmatic children.In addition to the family environment, the teenager's environment can have an impact on his or her asthma. By becoming involved in their community, adolescents are likely to face a variety of adverse situations (violence, poverty, discrimination, etc.). Thus, in a cross-sectional study of a sample of 61 African-American adolescents, high cumulative stress (poverty, neighbourhood stress, school stress, peer pressure, conflict between the adolescent and his parents) was also associated with deterioration in quality of life, reduced asthma control and visits to asthma emergency departments [98]. Given the high rate of co-morbid anxiety and depression in adolescents with asthma, regular screening of psychological status and family functioning to identify families at risk is recommended [85]. Moreover, in its recent guidelines, the American Academy of Pediatrics recommends universal screening for depression for all children over the age of 12 [99].For their part, health systems should develop programmes to make parents and young people aware of the high risk of anxiety and depressive disorders in adolescents with asthma, and develop anxiety and depression treatment programmes for these young people [85].In our series, psychological screening was carried out in only 14 cases (28%). Anxiety and depressive disorders were found in three asthmatic adolescents (21.4%). Anxiety and depressive disorders were observed in mothers in two cases (14.3%).

D. Respiratory function :

DRE is of little value during an exacerbation. It would confirm the obstructive syndrome and chest distension. However, they are essential in the intercritical period. It is of diagnostic and therapeutic value in monitoring asthma control, and also prognostic [100]. Intercritical obstruction, even in the absence of clinical perception, prompts the initiation or adjustment of background treatment.The measurement of PEF is a very useful adjunct to the measurement of bronchial obstruction in the clinic or at home [100]. PEF measurement is even more useful in certain subgroups of patients with a poor perception of their symptoms [3].Circadian variations of more than 20% in PEF indicate unstable asthma. The extent of the fall in PEF during an exacerbation and the evaluation of the response after the administration of □2-adrenergic improve management at home [100].According to Kamps et al [101], PEF monitoring is not necessary in the majority of children with asthma. Education is the most important component of asthma self-management. In our study, a decrease in intercritical PEF (<80% of theoretical value) was associated with poor asthma control in adolescents (p=0.018). On the other hand, an obstructive ventilatory disorder on intercritical EFR was not correlated with the level of asthma control (p=0.76).

E. Therapeutic characteristics :

I. Treatment :

ICS represent the first line of background treatment for asthma. Their efficacy in reducing asthma mortality, asthma symptoms and ventilatory function has been widely demonstrated [102].BLDAs act synergistically with ICSs. Corticosteroids also prevent possible desensitisation of beta2-mimetic receptors (tachyphylaxis). In a multicentre, randomised, double-blind study, 11679 patients with moderate to severe persistent asthma (age □ 12 years) were assigned to receive either fluticasone with salmeterol or fluticasone alone for 26 weeks. Patients receiving the fluticasone-salmeterol combination had a 21% lower risk of severe asthma exacerbations compared with the fluticasone alone group [103].

According to GINA 2018 [7], the use of BLDAs in combination with ICSs is from tier 3 of treatment.In our study, 96% of patients were started on ICS. Combination ICS with BLDA was used in 28% of cases. The choice of background treatment (ICS or ICS plus BLDA) had no effect on asthma control (p=0.71).

II. Technique for using the inhalation device :

Inhalation technique is generally poor in asthmatic children [104]. The same applies to adults [105].Poor inhalation technique can lead to poor treatment delivery, which can reduce the effectiveness of the treatment [104]. Several studies have reported a significant link between poor inhalation technique and poor asthma control [104,105,106]. The greater the number of technical errors, the poorer the asthma control [105].

According to Manriquez et al [107], the most common error noted in asthmatic children was failure to perform a 10-second apnea after inhalation. In a prospective cross-sectional study of 113 asthmatic children aged between 2 and 16 years hospitalised for asthma exacerbation, evaluation of the inhalation technique using an inhalation chamber showed that 42% of participants missed at least one essential step. The results were better when an inhalation chamber with a mask was used rather than a mouthpiece [108].

In a review of the literature by Gillette et al [104], all but one study indicated that communication was associated with better inhalation technique, and the more instruction the child received the better the technique. It's not enough to ask children if they're using their inhalers correctly. It is essential that healthcare providers ask children to demonstrate their inhalation technique at every consultation [109].

Similarly, interventions in schools involving the teaching of inhalation technique showed an improvement in technique over a 12-month period [110].

In our study, inhaler technique was assessed in 35 patients (70%). Although inhalation technique was not statistically related to asthma control (p=0.11), it was good in 94.3% of cases, demonstrating that the education given to patients during consultations was effective.

III. Therapeutic compliance :

In our series, poor compliance with medication was found in 44% of cases and was correlated with asthma control (p=0.002; OR=6.42 [1.86-22.2]). In multivariate analysis, poor compliance was the only factor associated with poor asthma control (p=0.011).

In asthmatic children, compliance is generally inadequate, at around 50% [111]. Adherence is even lower in adolescents [112]. Adolescents use asthma preventive treatment less frequently than children and adults with asthma.

The correlation between compliance and asthma control has been established in several studies. In a cross-sectional study of 1410 asthmatic children aged 6 to 14 years, compliance was significantly associated with asthma control (p=0.0005). Sixty-five per cent of children with controlled asthma were compliant [113]. In another prospective study involving 106 asthmatic children, McQuaid et al [114] established a negative relationship between therapeutic non-compliance and asthma control.A multivariate analysis, based on data from 10749 patients (adults and children), showed that the probability of having optimal asthma control was significantly higher in compliant patients than in non-compliant patients (OR=1.6; 95% CI [1.5; 1.8]) [115].

Compliance is not related to the severity of asthma. In a study of 433 children seen in emergency departments for asthma exacerbations, the level of compliance was the same as in the previous study. regardless of the severity of the asthma [116]. Barriers to compliance in adolescents include a negative attitude towards carers [117], reluctance to take medication in the presence of peers, and denial of the consequences of non-adherence to treatment [118].

In a cross-sectional study involving 126 adolescents with asthma aged 13 to 21 years, the most frequently cited obstacle to adherence to treatment was a negative attitude towards doctors and medication (63%), followed by forgetting to take the treatment (53%), then denial of the disease (50%). This study also identified lack of self-efficacy as the most influential psychosocial factor predicting non-adherence to treatment [119].

Lack of information about asthma medications and false beliefs also contribute to poor compliance [120]. Other treatment-related factors can affect compliance: confusion between immediate-acting treatment and long-term preventive treatment [121], poor understanding of the role of inhaled corticosteroid treatment [122] and fear of the side-effects of inhaled corticosteroids and bronchodilators [121].

Poor compliance may also be linked to the difficulty of using inhalation systems and the sometimes high cost of treatment [123]. On the other hand, good communication between doctor and patient is necessary to ensure patient compliance with treatment. However, communication with adolescents is particularly difficult [124]. The doctor must therefore develop his or her own techniques of active listening and mutual participation, and the questions asked must be open and permissive [125].

Decisions should not be dictated but negotiated with the adolescent so that they are accepted. In a randomised study of 2509 patients, including 721 children, the main determinants of compliance were the quality of the explanation of the treatment regimen, the time devoted to the consultation, the patient's feeling of being involved in the choice of treatment, and the regularity of follow-up [126]. Understanding how adolescents function is essential to improving compliance. Neuroscientists have paid a great deal of attention to the adolescent brain in recent years, in particular in an attempt to understandwhy this period of life is characterised by risk-taking and risk-taking behaviour sub-optimal decision-making. Neuroscience attributes this behaviour in adolescents to an imbalance between the rapid maturation of the limbic system responsible for impulsivity and the slower maturation of the prefrontal cortex responsible for control and long-term vision [127].The influence of the limbic system predominates when choosing an immediate reward, while activation of the prefrontal regions is more important when choosing a longer-term reward. Adolescence is therefore a period during which disease-modifying therapy is very unlikely to be taken, as it offers no short-term benefits, while its long-term benefits are not perceived. In the Cochrane systematic review published in 2014 on interventions to improve medication adherence, the authors concluded that the methods used to improve adherence in chronic diseases were mostly complex and not very effective [128]. In fact, these interventions required adolescents to have better control over their compliance, by educating them intensively, involving them in behavioural therapies and reminding them daily of the need for treatment. Their ineffectiveness could be linked to an error in targeting: the prefrontal regions are not yet mature in adolescents.

On the contrary, given the predominance of limbic system activity over prefrontal regions in adolescence, the greatest hopes of improving compliance now lie in neuro-technological interventions targeting this limbic system. One such approach has been applied to adolescents and young adults with cancer, using a video game called "Re-Mission" [129]. This action game put the player in the shoes of a nanobot exploring the bodies of young patients with haematological malignancies and solid cancers. The player's objective is to destroy cancer cells and opportunistic infections, and to manage the side effects of chemotherapy. A multicentre study conducted in the United States and Canada compared the use of this video game, played freely for 3 months, by 375 young people aged 13 to 29, with the use of a commercial game (Indiana Jones) played freely for the same period. Re-Mission" players were more compliant with chemotherapy and antibiotic prophylaxis. With regard to unintentional non-adherence (forgetfulness), the development of new technologies has made it possible to devise new solutions to improve adolescent compliance. A study carried out specifically on adolescents with asthma included 89 participants aged 12 to 17 randomised into two groups, one receiving short text message (SMS) reminders at the times when treatment should be taken, and the other not [130]. It showed an improvement in self-reported compliance in the group receiving the SMS.

F. Effects of asthma :

I. School :

On average, asthma affects one in ten schoolchildren. School absenteeism is common, reflecting poor control of asthma [131].In the United States, more than 10 million school days are missed each year because of asthma [132].In the AIRE study [133], 42.7% of asthmatic children in Europe missed school at least once a year. In a randomised telephone survey conducted in the United States (35 states), 51% of children had missed at least one day of school because of asthma in the previous 12 months. The causes of asthma-related school absenteeism were: uncontrolled asthma, frequent use of urgent care, financial barriers to accessing care and the presence of mould in the home [134]. Poorly controlled asthma, which leads to absenteeism, is a factor in children falling behind at school [131]. This delay can also be explained by sleep disorders, which are more frequent in asthmatic children than in their healthy peers. Sleep disturbance is the cause of memory and concentration problems [135], and reduces school performance [136].Neglected or accepted, the delay in schooling will be responsible for too early a career choice, often inappropriate for asthmatic children, leading to manual occupations, which are much more likely to cause occupational asthma than other professions [131].In our study, difficulties at school were only observed in the uncontrolled group (31.8%), and the association with poor asthma control was significant (p=0.002).

II. Physical activity :

Children and adolescents with asthma should be encouraged to engage in regular physical activity. One of the aims of long-term asthma management is to enable patients to maintain a normal level of activity [7].

Studies to determine whether children and adolescents with asthma are less active than their healthy peers have produced contradictory results.Some studies have found no association between reduced physical activity and asthma [137,138]. On the other hand, in other studies this association was observed only in cases of exercise-induced bronchospasm [139], recent hospitalisation [138] or obesity [140].

In a cross-sectional study of 55 children with newly diagnosed asthma (aged 6 to 14 years) and 154 healthy control children, asthmatic children were initially started on inhaled corticosteroids. After a one-year follow-up, improvement in asthma control was associated with a significant increase in total daily activity of 2.8 hours per week compared with healthy controls (p<0.001) [141].The practice of sport, long prohibited or inadvisable in asthmatic children, is now a therapeutic option, with both physiological and psychological benefits. It reduces exertional dyspnoea, reduces exertional asthma attacks and improves the child's socialisation with peers of the same age [131]. In our study, limitation of physical activity was significantly correlated with poor asthma control (p=0.005). In particular, it was not reported by adolescents in the control group.

CONCLUSIONS

Asthma is the most common chronic disease in the paediatric population. The prevalence of asthma in adolescents aged 13-14 is estimated at 13.7%, compared with 11.6% in children aged 6-7. Tunisia is one of the high-prevalence countries [1]. Adolescence is a period of transition from childhood to adulthood, characterised by intense developmental, emotional and psychosocial changes. Asthmatic children's quality of life depends on how well their asthma is controlled.The aims of our study were to analyse the clinical, spirometric and therapeutic characteristics of asthma in adolescents, and to identify the factors influencing asthma control in this population. The study was conducted in the Paediatric Pneumology Department of the Abderrahmane Mami Pneumo- phtisiology Centre in Ariana over a five-year period (2015-2019).This was a retrospective, cross-sectional, descriptive study involving 50 adolescents with asthma. The patients were divided into a controlled group of 28 and an uncontrolled group of 22. The assessment of asthma control was based on GINA 2018. The mean age of patients included in the study was 12.8 years, with a mean duration of disease of 8.3 years. The sex ratio was 1.8.

In the control group, the mean age was 13 years, with a sex ratio of 1.8. The mean duration of the disease was 7.9 years. Exposure to passive smoking was observed in 46.4% of cases. Dampness in the home was reported in 32.1% of cases. Obesity was noted in three adolescents (10.7%). Asthma was allergic in 52.4% of cases. No delay in schooling or reduction in sporting activity was reported. Psychological evaluation was carried out in 6 adolescents and showed anxiety or depression in 3 cases.In terms of function, a moderate decrease in PEF was noted in 12% of adolescents. Spirometry showed an obstructive ventilatory disorder in 60.7% of cases. In terms of treatment, inhaled corticosteroids were used by 92.9% of adolescents. Compliance was good in 75% of cases.

In the uncontrolled group, the mean age was 12.7 years, with a sex ratio of 1.8. The mean duration of the disease was 8.7 years. Half the adolescents were exposed to passive smoking. Socio-economic conditions were considered poor in 13.7% of cases, and dampness in the home was reported in 63.6% of cases. There was no obesity in this group. Asthma was allergic in 58.8% of cases. Delayed school attendance and reduced sporting activity were reported in 31.8% and 27.3% of cases respectively. Psychological assessment was carried out in eight adolescents, and showed depression in one case. In terms of function, a moderate to severe reduction in PEF was noted in 42.9% of adolescents. Spirometry, performed on 20 adolescents, showed obstructive ventilatory disorders in 65% of cases. In terms of treatment, all patients used inhaled corticosteroids, with long-acting beta-2 mimetics being used in combination in 31.8% of adolescents. Compliance was poor in 68.2% of cases.

The factors identified in our study as contributing to poor asthma control were :

- The presence of dampness in the home (OR=3.69),

- a reduction in intercritical peak expiratory flow (OR=5.5),

- poor compliance with treatment (OR=6.42).

In a multivariate study, the only factor identified as contributing to poor asthma control in adolescents was poor compliance with treatment (p=0.011). Poor asthma control was significantly correlated with difficulties at school (p=0.002) and a reduction in sporting activity (p=0.005) observed in adolescents.The complexity of managing asthma in adolescence is linked to a number of specific factors, including developmental problems and risk behaviours, more frequent psychological disorders, particularly anxiety and depression, especially in severe forms, and denial of the disease. In addition, the desire The asthmatic teenager's desire to be no different, and peer pressure, only exacerbate the lack of adherence to treatment. Added to this are cultural problems and, in particular, misconceptions about disease-modifying therapy. To improve adherence to treatment and thus promote asthma control in adolescents, we suggest :

- Emphasise to the teenager and his or her parents the need not to interrupt the disease-modifying treatment, explaining the chronic nature of the disease.

- Psychological assessment should be strengthened and made a systematic part of the follow-up of asthmatic adolescents. This assessment should be repeated if asthma becomes more severe.

- Involve the social worker in monitoring the asthmatic teenager, so that intra-family problems, particularly conflict situations and financial problems, can be detected early and remedied in time.

- Improving the care of asthmatic adolescents in the school environment through educational programmes targeting both teachers, to improve their knowledge of asthma and thus provide better support for patients in their school lives, and above all peers, whose preponderant role in asthmatic adolescents' compliance with treatment has been highlighted in various epidemiological studies.

REFERENCES

1. Pearce N, Aït-Khaled N, Beasley R, Mallol J, Keil U, Mitchell E et al. Worldwide trends in the prevalence of asthma symptoms: phase III of the International Study of Asthma and Allergies in Childhood (ISAAC). Thorax. 2007;62:758-66.

2. Rancé F, Bataille H, Brémont F, Rittié JL, Dutau G, Didier A. Adult prognosis of adolescent asthma. Rev Mal Respir. 2000;17:1089-93.

3. How should asthma control be defined and on what basis should it be assessed? Recommendations for the medical follow-up of adult and adolescent asthma patients. Rev Mal Respir. 2005;22:23-44.

4. De Blic J, Deschildre A. Monitoring asthmatic children: definition and measurement tools. Rev Mal Respir. 2008;25:695-704.

5. Schmier JK, Manjunath R, Halpern MT, Jones ML, Thompson K, Diette GB. The impact of inadequately controlled asthma in urban children on quality of life and productivity. Ann Allergy Asthma Immunol. 2007;98:245-51.

6. Sullivan SD, Rasouliyan L, Russo PA, Kamath T, Chipps BE. Extent, patterns, and burden of uncontrolled disease in severe or difficult-to-treat asthma. Allergy. 2007;62:126-33.

7. Global Initiative for Asthma. Global Strategy for Asthma Management and Prevention, 2018. Available from: www.ginasthma.org.

8. World Health Organization. Young people's health-a challenge for society. Report of a WHO Study Group on Young People and "Health for All by the Year 2000". Geneva: WHO; 1986. Technical Report Series, No. 731.

9. Carsin A, Pham-Thi N. Asthmatic exacerbations: paediatric specificities (apart from treatment). Rev Mal Respir. 2011;28(10):1322-8.

10. Martinez FD, Wright AL, Taussig LM, Holberg CJ, Halonen M, Morgan WJ. Asthma and wheezing in the first six years of life. N Engl J Med. 1995;332:133- 8.

11. Smit LAM, Bouzigon E, Pin I, Siroux V, Monier F, Aschard H. 17q21 variants modify the association between early respiratory infections and asthma. Eur Respir J. 2010;36:57-64.

12. Just J, Bourgoin-Heck M, Amat F. Clinical phenotypes in asthma during childhood. Clin Exp Allergy. 2017;47:848-55.

13. Zein JG, Erzurum SC. Asthma is different in women. Curr Allergy Asthma Rep. 2015;15(6):28.

14. DeBoer MD, Phillips BR, Mauger DT, Zein J, Erzurum SC, Fitzpatrick AM et al. Effects of endogenous sex hormones on lung function and symptom control in adolescents with asthma. BMC Pulm Med. 2018;18(1):58.

15. Schatz M, Clark S, Camargo CA. Sex differences in the presentation and course of asthma hospitalizations. Chest. 2006;129(1):50-5.

16. Varraso R, Siroux V, Maccario J, Pin I, Kauffmann F. Asthma severity is associated with body mass index and early menarche in women. Am J Respir Crit Care Med.

2005;171(4):334-9.

17. Sears MR, Greene JM, Willan AR, Wiecek EM, Taylor DR, Flannery EM et al. A longitudinal, population-based, cohort study of childhood asthma followed to adulthood. N Engl J Med. 2003;349(15):1414-22.

18. El Ftouh M, Yassine N, Benkheder A, Bouacha H, Nafti S, Taright S et al. Paediatric asthma in North Africa: the Asthma Insights and Reality in the Maghreb (AIRMAG) study. Respir Med. 2009; 103 Suppl 2:S21-S29.

19. Antunes H, Precioso J, Araújo AC, Machado JC, Samorinha S, Rocha V et al. Prevalence of secondhand smoke exposure in asthmatic children at home and in the car: A cross-sectional study. Rev Port Pneumol. 2016;22(4):190-5.

20. Merianos AL, Jandarov RA, Mahabee-Gittens EM. Association of secondhand smoke exposure with asthma symptoms, medication use, and healthcare utilization among asthmatic adolescents. J Asthma. 2019;56(4):369-79.

21. Neophytou AM, Oh SS, White MJ, Mak ACY, Hu D, Huntsman S et al. Secondhand smoke exposure and asthma outcomes among African-American and Latino children with asthma. Thorax. 2018;73:1041-8.

22. De Blic J, Boucot I, Pribil C, Robert R, Huas D, Marguet C. Control of asthma in children: still unacceptable? A French cross-sectional study. Respir Med. 2009;103:1383-91.

23. Jing W, Wang W, Liu Q. Passive smoking induces pediatric asthma by affecting the balance of Treg/Th17 cells. Pediatr Res. 2019;85(4):469-76.

24. Halterman JS, Szilagyi PG, Yoos L, Conn KM, Kaczorowski JM, Holzhauer RJ et al. Benefits of a school-based asthma treatment program in the absence of secondhand smoke exposure: results of a randomized clinical trial. Arch Pediatr Adolesc Med. 2004;158:460-7.

25. Howrylak JA, Spanier AJ, Huang B, Peake RWA, Kellogg MD, Sauers H et al. Cotinine in children admitted for asthma and readmission. Pediatrics. 2014;133(2):e355-62.

26. Deschildre A, Pin I, Gueorguieva I, De Blic J. Asthma and obesity: what is the relationship in children? Arch Pediatr. 2009;16(8):1166-74.

27. Von Mutius E, Schwartz J, Neas LM, Dockery D, Weiss ST. Relation of body mass index to asthma and atopy in children: the National Health and Nutrition Examination Study III. Thorax. 2001;56(11):835-8.

28. Castro-Rodriguez JA, Holberg CJ, Morgan WJ, Wright AL, Martinez FD. Increased incidence of asthmalike symptoms in girls who become overweight or obese during the school years. Am J Respir Crit Care Med. 2001;163(6):1344-9.

29. Sbarbati A. Obesity and inflammation: evidence for an elementary lesion. Pediatrics. 2006;117(1):220-3.

30. Shore SA. Obesity and asthma: lessons from animal models. J Appl Physiol. 2007;102:516-28.

31. Shore SA. Obesity and asthma: possible mechanisms. J Allergy Clin Immunol. 2008;121:1087-93.

32. Parameswaran K, Todd DC, Soth M. Altered respiratory physiology in obesity. Can Respir J. 2006;13(4):203-10.

33. Sonnenschein-van der Voort AMM, Howe LD, Granell R, Duijts L, Sterne JAC, Tilling K et al. Influence of childhood growth on asthma and lung function in adolescence. J Allergy Clin Immunol. 2015;135:1435-43.

34. Hayes Jr D, Jhaveri MA, Mannino DM, Strawbridge H, Temprano J. The effect of mold sensitization and humidity upon allergic asthma. Clin Respir J. 2013;7:135-44.

35. Williamson IJ, Martin CJ, McGill G, Monie RDH, Fennerty AG. Damp housing and asthma: a case-control study. Thorax. 1997;52:229-34.

36. Nicolai T, Illi S, Von Mutius E. Effect of dampness at home in childhood on bronchial hyperreactivity in adolescence. Thorax. 1998;53:1035-40.

37. Apelberg BJ, Aoki Y, Jaakkola JJK. Systematic review: Exposure to pets and risk of asthma and asthma-like symptoms. J Allergy Clin Immunol. 2001;107:455- 60.

38. Strachan DP, Carey IM. Home environment and severe asthma in adolescence: a population based case-control study. BMJ. 1995;311:1053-6.

39. Sarpong SB, Karrison T. Sensitization to indoor allergens and the risk for asthma hospitalization in children. Ann Allergy Asthma Immunol. 1997;79(5):455-9.

40. Custovic A, Murray CS, Gore RB, Woodcock A. Controlling indoor allergens. Ann Allergy Asthma Immunol. 2002;88(5):432-41.

41. Adler NE, Boyce T, Chesney MA, Folkman S, Syme SL. Socioeconomic inequalities in health. No easy solution. JAMA. 1993;269:3140-5.

42. Chen E, Matthews KA, Boyce WT. Socioeconomic differences in children's health: how and why do these relationships change with age? Psychol Bull. 2002;128(2):295-329.

43. Miller JE. The effects of race/ethnicity and income on early childhood asthma prevalence and health care use. Am J Public Health. 2000;90:428-30.

44. Persky VW, Slezak J, Contreras A, Becker L, Hernandez E, Ramakrishnan V et al. Relationships of race and socioeconomic status with prevalence, severity, and symptoms of asthma in Chicago school children. Ann Allergy Asthma Immunol. 1998;81:266-71.

45. Chen E, Fisher EB, Bacharier LB, Strunk RC. Socioeconomic status, stress, and immune markers in adolescents with asthma. Psychosom Med. 2003;65:984- 92.

46. Chen E, Hanson MD, Paterson LQ, Griffin MJ, Walker HA, Miller GE. J Allergy Clin Immunol. 2006;117:1014-20.

47. Kang DH, Coe CL, McCarthy DO, Jarjour NN, Kelly EA, Rodriguez RR et al. Cytokine profiles of stimulated blood lymphocytes in asthmatic and healthy adolescents across the school year. J Interferon Cytokine Res. 1997;17(8):481- 7.

48. Liu LY, Coe CL, Swenson CA, Kelly EA, Kita H, Busse WW. School examinations enhance airway inflammation to antigen challenge. Am J Respir Crit Care Med. 2002;165:1062-7.

49. Wright RJ, Finn P, Contreras JP, Cohen S, Wright RO, Staudenmayer J et al. Chronic

caregiver stress and IgE expression, allergen-induced proliferation, and cytokine profiles in a birth cohort predisposed to atopy. J Allergy Clin Immunol. 2004;113(6):1051-7.

50. Fries E, Hesse J, Hellhammer J, Hellhammer DH. A new view on hypocortisolism. Psychoneuroendocrinology. 2005;30:1010-6.

51. Williams DR, Sternthal M, Wright RJ. Social determinants: taking the social context of asthma seriously. Pediatrics. 2009;123 Suppl 3:S174-S184.

52. Sporik R, Holgate ST, Platts-Mills TA, Cogswell JJ. Exposure to house-dust mite allergen (Der p I) and the development of asthma in childhood. A prospective study. N Engl J Med. 1990;323:502-7.

53. Katz LF, Kling JR, Liebman JB. Moving to opportunity in Boston: early results of a randomized mobility experiment. Q J Econ. 2001;116(2):607-54.

54. Chen E, Shalowitz MU, Story RE, Ehrlich KB, Levine CS, Hayen R et al. Dimensions of socioeconomic status and childhood asthma outcomes: evidence for distinct behavioral and biological associations. Psychosom Med. 2016;78(9):1043-52.

55. Patel MR, Brown RW, Clark NM. Perceived parent financial burden and asthma outcomes in low-income, urban children. J Urban Health. 2013;90:329-42.

56. Kozyrskyj AL, Mustard CA, Simons FE. Inhaled corticosteroids in childhood asthma: income differences in use. Pediatr Pulmonol. 2003;36:241-7.

57. Kozyrskyj AL, Mustard CA, Simons FE. Socioeconomic status, drug insurance benefits, and new prescriptions for inhaled corticosteroids in schoolchildren with asthma. Arch Pediatr Adolesc Med. 2001;155:1219-24.

58. Gray WN, Netz M, McConville A, Fedele D, Wagoner ST, Schaefer MR. Medication adherence in pediatric asthma: a systematic review of the literature. Pediatr Pulmonol. 2018;53:668-84.

59. Jonasson G, Carlsen K, Mowinckel P. Asthma drug adherence in a long term clinical trial. Arch Dis Child. 2000;83:330-3.

60. Delacourt C. Place of inhaled corticosteroid therapy in the prevention of bronchial remodelling. Controversy: against. Rev Fr Allergol Immunol Clin. 2003;43:442-5.

61. Vidal A, Ubilla C, Duffau G. Control de asthma en adolescentes : Assessment of disease control among asthmatic adolescents. Rev Med Chile. 2008;136:859- 66.

62. Bergström S, Sundell K, Hedlin G. Adolescents with asthma: consequences of transition from paediatric to adult healthcare. Respir Med. 2010;104:180-7.

63. Malmström K, Pitkäranta A, Carpen O, Pelkonen A, Malmberg LP, Turpeinen M et al. Human rhinovirus in bronchial epithelium of infants with recurrent respiratory symptoms. J Allergy Clin Immunol. 2006;118:591-6.

64. Hedlin G, Bush A, Carlsen KL, Wennergren G, De Benedictis FM, Melén E et al. Problematic severe asthma in children, not one problem but many: a GA2LEN initiative. Eur Respir J. 2010;36:196-201.

65. Barton CA, McKenzie DP, Walters EH, Abramson MJ. Interactions between

psychosocial problems and management of asthma: who is at risk of dying? J Asthma. 2005;42:249-56.

66. De Blic J, Boucot I, Pribil C, Huas D, Godard P. Level of asthma control in children in general practice in France: results of the ER'ASTHME study. Arch Pediatr. 2007;14:1069-75.

67. Cockcroft DW, Swystun VA. Asthma control versus asthma severity. J Allergy Clin Immunol. 1996;98:1016-8.

68. Tsao SM, Ko YK, Chen MZ, Chiu MH, Lin CS, Lin MS et al. A survey of allergic rhinitis in Taiwanese asthma patients. J Microbiol Immunol Infect. 2011;44(2):139-43.

69. De Groot EP, Nijkamp A, Duiverman EJ, Brand PLP. Allergic rhinitis is associated with poor asthma control in children with asthma. Thorax. 2012;67:582-7.

70. Bousquet J, Schünemann HJ, Samolinski B, Demoly P, Baena-Cagnani CE, Bachert C et al. Allergic Rhinitis and its Impact on Asthma (ARIA): achievements in 10 years and future needs. J Allergy Clin Immunol. 2012;130:1049-62.

71. Ponte EV, Franco R, Nascimento HF, Souza-Machado A, Cunha S, Barreto ML et al. Lack of control of severe asthma is associated with co-existence of moderate- to-severe rhinitis. Allergy. 2008;63:564-9.

72. Magnan A, Meunier JP, Saugnac C, Gasteau J, Neukirch F. Frequency and impact of allergic rhinitis in asthma patients in everyday general medical practice: a French observational cross-sectional study. Allergy. 2008;63:292-8.

73. Peroni DG, Piacentini GL, Ceravolo R, Boner AL. Difficult asthma: possible association with rhinosinusitis. Pediatr Allergy Immunol. 2007;18 Suppl 18:25- 7.

74. Crystal-Peaters J, Neslusan C, Crown WH, Torres A. Treating allergic rhinitis in patients with comorbid asthma: the risk of asthma-related hospitalizations and emergency department visits. J Allergy Clin Immunol. 2002;109:57-62.

75. Yu CL, Huang WT, Wang CM. Treatment of allergic rhinitis reduces acute asthma exacerbation risk among asthmatic children aged 2-18 years. J Microbiol Immunol Infect. 2019;52:991-9.

76. Pin I, Pilenko C, Chatain P, Llerena C, Bost M. Environnement et asthme de l'enfant : controverses et jusqu'où aller? Arch Pediatr. 2004;11 Suppl 2:S93- S97.

77. Siroux V, Oryszczyn MP, Varraso R, Le Moual N, Bousquet J, Charpin D et al. Environmental factors in severe asthma and allergy: results of the EGEA study. Rev Mal Respir. 2007;24:599-608.

78. Carroll W, Lenney W, Child F, Strange RC, Jones PW, Whyte MK et al. Asthma severity and atopy: how clear is the relationship? Arch Dis Child. 2006;91:405- 9.

79. Turner S, Eaton T, Rowe J, Suriyaarachchi D, Serralha M, Holt BJ et al. Early- onset atopy is associated with enhanced lymphocyte cytokine responses in 11- year-old children. Clin Exp Allergy. 2007;37:371-80.

80. Siroux V, Oryszczyn MP, Paty E, Kauffmann F, Pison C, Vervloet D et al. Relationships of allergic sensitization, total immunoglobulin E and blood eosinophils to asthma severity in children of the EGEA Study. Clin Exp Allergy. 2003;33:746-51.

81. Lu Y, Mak KK, Van Bever HPS, Ng TP, Mak A, Ho RCM. Prevalence of anxiety and depressive symptoms in adolescents with asthma: a meta-analysis and meta-regression. Pediatr Allergy Immunol. 2012;23:707-15.

82. Bender BG. Risk taking, depression, adherence, and symptom control in adolescents and young adults with asthma. Am J Respir Crit Care Med. 2006;173:953-7.

83. Dudeney J, Sharpe L, Jaffe A, Jones EB, Hunt C. Anxiety in youth with asthma: a meta-analysis. Pediatr Pulmonol. 2017;52:1121-9.

84. Bender B, Zhang L. Negative affect, medication adherence, and asthma control in children. J Allergy Clin Immunol. 2008;122:490-5.

85. Katon W, Lozano P, Russo J, McCauley E, Richardson L, Bush T. The prevalence of DSM-IV anxiety and depressive disorders in youth with asthma compared to controls. J Adolesc Health. 2007;41(5):455-63.

86. Chen E, Miller GE. Stress and inflammation in exacerbations of asthma. Brain Behav Immun. 2007;21(8):993-9.

87. Miller GE, Chen E. Life stress and diminished expression of genes encoding glucocorticoid receptor and beta2-adrenergic receptor in children with asthma. Proc Natl Acad Sci U S A. 2006;103(14):5496-501.

88. Brehm JM, Ramratnam SK, Tse SM, Croteau-Chonka DC, Pino-Yanes M, Rosas-Salazar C, et al. Stress and bronchodilator response in children with asthma. Am J Respir Crit Care Med. 2015;192(1):47-56.

89. Chen E, Hanson MD, Paterson LQ, Griffin MJ, Walker HA, Miller GE. Socioeconomic status and inflammatory processes in childhood asthma: the role of psychological stress. J Allergy Clin Immunol. 2006;117(5):1014-20.

90. Landeo-Gutierrez J, Forno E, Miller GE, Celedón JC. Exposure to violence, psychosocial stress, and asthma. Am J Respir Crit Care Med. 2020;201(8):917- 22.

91. Ohno I. Neuropsychiatry phenotype in asthma: psychological stress-induced alterations of the neuroendocrine-immune system in allergic airway inflammation. Allergol Int. 2017;66S:S2-S8.

92. Oren E, Gerald L, Stern DA, Martinez FD, Wright AL. Self-reported stressful life events during adolescence and subsequent asthma: a longitudinal study. J Allergy Clin Immunol Pract. 2017;5(2):427-34.

93. Chen E, Strunk RC, Bacharier LB, Chan M, Miller GE. Socioeconomic status associated with exhaled nitric oxide responses to acute stress in children with asthma. Brain Behav Immun. 2010;24(3):444-50.

94. Shankar M, Fagnano M, Blaakman SW, Rhee H, Halterman JS. Depressive symptoms among urban adolescents with asthma: a focus for providers. Acad Pediatr. 2019;19(6):608-14.

95. Wood BL, Lim J, Miller BD, Cheah PA, Simmens S, Stern T et al. Family emotional climate, depression, emotional triggering of asthma, and disease severity in pediatric asthma: examination of pathways of effect. J Pediatr Psychol. 2007;32:542-51.

96. Kaugars AS, Klinnert MD, Bender BG. Family influences on pediatric asthma. J Pediatr Psychol. 2004;29(7):475-91.

97. Wolf JM, Miller GE, Chen E. Parent psychological states predict changes in inflammatory markers in children with asthma and healthy children. Brain Behav Immun. 2008;22(4):433-41.

98. Miadich SA, Everhart RS, Greenlee J, Winter MA. The impact of cumulative stress on asthma outcomes among urban adolescents. J Adolesc. 2020;80:254- 63.

99. Zuckerbrot RA, Cheung A, Jensen PS, Stein REK, Laraque D. Guidelines for adolescent depression in primary care (GLAD-PC): part I. Practice preparation, identification, assessment, and initial management. Pediatrics. 2018;141(3):e20174081.

100.De Blic J. Asthma in children and young children. EMC-Pediatrics. 2016;11(1):1- 15.

101.Kamps AW, Brand PL. Education, self-management and home peak flow monitoring in childhood asthma. Paediatr Respir Rev. 2001;2(2):165-9.

102.Boushey HA. Effects of inhaled corticosteroids on the consequences of asthma. J Allergy Clin Immunol. 1998;102(4):S5-S16.

103.Stempel DA, Raphiou IH, Kral KM, Yeakey AM, Emmett AH, Prazma CM, et al. Serious asthma events with fluticasone plus salmeterol versus fluticasone alone. N Engl J Med. 2016;374(19):1822-30.

104.Gillette C, Rockich-Winston N, Kuhn JA, Flesher S, Shepherd M. Inhaler technique in children with asthma: a systematic review. Acad Pediatr. 2016;16(7):605-15.

105.Giraud V, Roche N. Misuse of corticosteroid metered-dose inhaler is associated with decreased asthma stability. Eur Respir J. 2002;19:246-51.

106.Giraud V. Evaluation of asthma control: a clinical practice audit. Rev Mal Respir. 2005;22 :219-26.

107.Manríquez P, Acuña AM, Muñoz L, Reyes A. Study of inhaler technique in asthma patients: differences between pediatric and adult patients. J Bras Pneumol. 2015;41(5):405-9.

108.Samady W, Rodriguez VA, Gupta R, Palac H, Karamanis M, Press VG. Critical errors in inhaler technique among children hospitalized with asthma. J Hosp Med. 2019;14(6):361-5.

109.Alexander DS, Geryk L, Arrindell C, DeWalt DA, Weaver MA, Sleath B, et al. Are children with asthma overconfident that they are using their inhalers correctly? J Asthma. 2016;53(1):107-12.

110.Geryk LL, Roberts CA, Carpenter DM. A systematic review of school-based interventions that include inhaler technique education. Respir Med. 2017;132:21-30.

111.De Blic J. Therapeutic compliance in asthmatic children. Rev Mal Respir. 2007;24:419- 25.

112.Kit BK, Simon AE, Ogden CL, Akinbami LJ. Trends in preventive asthma medication use among children and adolescents, 1988-2008. Pediatrics. 2012;129(1):62-9.

113.Tantisira KG, Litonjua AA, Weiss ST, Fuhlbrigge AL. Association of body mass with pulmonary function in the Childhood Asthma Management Program (CAMP). Thorax.

2003;58:1036-41.

114.McQuaid EL, Kopel SJ, Klein RB, Fritz GK. Medication adherence in pediatric asthma: reasoning, responsibility, and behavior. J Pediatr Psychol. 2003;28:323-33.

115.Godard P, Huas D, Sobier B, Pribil C, Boucot I. ER'Asthme, asthma control in 16580 patients followed in general practice. Press Med. 2005;34:1351-7.

116.Scarfone RJ, Zorc JJ, Capraro GA. Patient self-management of acute asthma: adherence to national guidelines a decade later. Pediatrics. 2001;108:1332-8.

117.Cohen R, Franco K, Motlow F, Reznik M, Ozuah PO. Perceptions and attitudes of adolescents with asthma. J Asthma. 2003;40:207-11.

118.Rhee H, Wenzel J, Steeves RH. Adolescents' psychosocial experiences living with asthma: a focus group study. J Pediatr Health Care. 2007;21:99-107.

119.Rhee H, Belyea MJ, Ciurzynski S, Brasch J. Barriers to asthma self-management in adolescents: relationships to psychosocial factors. Pediatr Pulmonol. 2009;44(2):183-91.

120.Wamboldt FS, Bender BG, Rankin AE. Adolescent decision-making about use of inhaled asthma controller medication: results from focus groups with participants from a prior longitudinal study. J Asthma. 2011;48:741-50.

121.Payot F. Asthma in children: how to improve compliance. Arch Ped. 2006;13(6):540-3.

122.Farber HJ, Capra AM, Finkelstein JA, Lozano P, Quesenberry CP, Jensvold NG et al. Misunderstanding of asthma controller medications: association with nonadherence. J Asthma. 2003;40:17-25.

123.Walders N, Kopel SJ, Koinis-Mitchell D, McQuaid EL. Patterns of quick-relief and long-term controller medication use in pediatric asthma. J Pediatr. 2005;146:177-82.

124.De Benedictis D, Bush A. The challenge of asthma in adolescence. Pediatr Pulmonol. 2007;42:683-92.

125.Evans D. To help patients control asthma the clinician must be a good listener and teacher. Thorax. 1993;48:685-7.

126.Adams RJ, Weiss ST, Fuhlbrigge A. How and by whom care is delivered influences anti-inflammatory use in asthma: results of a national population survey. J Allergy Clin Immunol. 2003;112:445-50.

127.Casey BJ, Getz S, Galvan A. The adolescent brain. Dev Rev. 2008; 28:62-77.

128.Nieuwlaat R, Wilczynski N, Navarro T, Hobson N, Jeffery R, Keepanasseril A et al. Interventions for enhancing medication adherence. Cochrane Database Syst Rev. 2014;11:CD000011.

129.Kato PM, Cole SW, Bradlyn AS, et al. A video game improves behavioral outcomes in adolescents and young adults with cancer: a randomized trial. Pediatrics. 2008; 122 (2):e305-17.

130.Johnson KB, Patterson BL, Ho YX, Chen Q, Nian H, Davison CL, et al. The feasibility of text reminders to improve medication adherence in adolescents with asthma. J Am Med

Inform Assoc. 2016;23:449-55.

131.Karila C, Luc C, Dubus JC. The asthmatic child in the school environment: difficulties encountered, solutions envisaged.... Arch Pediatr. 2004;11 Suppl 2:S120-S123.

132.Akinbami LJ, Moorman JE, Liu X. Asthma prevalence, health care use, and mortality: United States, 2005-2009. Natl Health Stat Report. 2011;32:1-14.

133.Blanc FX, Postel-Vinay N, Boucot I, De Blic J, Scheinmann P. AIRE study: analysis of data collected from 753 asthmatic children in Europe. Rev Mal Respir. 2002;19 (5):585-92.

134.Hsu J, Qin X, Beavers SF, Mirabelli MC. Asthma-related school absenteeism, morbidity, and modifiable factors. Am J Prev Med 2016;51(1):23-32.

135.Stores G, Ellis AJ, Wiggs L, Crawford C, Thomson A. Sleep and psychological disturbance in nocturnal asthma. Arch Dis Child. 1998;78:413-9.

136.Diette GB, Markson L, Skinner EA, Nguyen TTH, Algatt-Bergstrom P, Wu AW. Nocturnal asthma in children affects school attendance, school performance, and parents' work attendance. Arch Pediatr Adolesc Med. 2000;154:923-8.

137.Cassim R, Koplin JJ, Dharmage SC, Senaratna BCV, Lodge CJ, Lowe AJ et al. The difference in amount of physical activity performed by children with and without asthma: a systematic review and meta-analysis. J Asthma. 2016;53:882-92.

138.Pike KC, Griffiths LJ, Dezateux C, Pearce A. Physical activity among children with asthma: cross-sectional analysis in the UK millennium cohort. Pediatr Pulmonol. 2019;54:962-9.

139.Van der Kamp MR, Thio BJ, Tabak M, Hermens HJ, Driessen JMM, Van der Palen JAM. Does exercise-induced bronchoconstriction affect physical activity patterns in asthmatic children? J Child Health Care. 2020;24:577-88.

140.Sousa AW, Cabral ALB, Martins MA, Carvalho CRF. Daily physical activity in asthmatic children with distinct severities. J Asthma. 2014;51:493-7.

141.Vahlkvist S, Inman MD, Pedersen S. Effect of asthma treatment on fitness, daily activity and body composition in children with asthma. Allergy. 2010;65:1464- 71.

APPENDICES

Appendix 1: Level of asthma control according to GINA 2018

Box 2-2. GINA assessment of asthma control in adults, adolescents and children 6–11 years

A. Asthma symptom control		Level of asthma symptom control		
In the past 4 weeks, has the patient had:		Well controlled	Partly controlled	Uncontrolled
• Daytime asthma symptoms more than twice/week?	Yes☐ No☐	None of these	1–2 of these	3–4 of these
• Any night waking due to asthma?	Yes☐ No☐			
• Reliever needed for symptoms* more than twice/week?	Yes☐ No☐			
• Any activity limitation due to asthma?	Yes☐ No☐			

B. Risk factors for poor asthma outcomes

Assess risk factors at diagnosis and periodically, particularly for patients experiencing exacerbations.

Measure FEV_1 at start of treatment, after 3–6 months of controller treatment to record the patient's personal best lung function, then periodically for ongoing risk assessment.

Having uncontrolled asthma symptoms is an important risk factor for exacerbations.[79]

Additional potentially modifiable risk factors for flare-ups (exacerbations), even in patients with few symptoms,[†] include:
- High SABA use[80] (with increased mortality if >1 x 200-dose canister/month[81])
- Inadequate ICS: not prescribed ICS; poor adherence;[82] incorrect inhaler technique[83]
- Low FEV_1, especially if <60% predicted[84,85]
- Higher bronchodilator reversibility[86,87]
- Major psychological or socioeconomic problems[88]
- Exposures: smoking;[85] allergen exposure if sensitized[85]
- Comorbidities: obesity;[89] chronic rhinosinusitis;[90] confirmed food allergy[91]
- Sputum or blood eosinophilia[92,93]
- Elevated FENO (in adults with allergic asthma taking ICS)[94]
- Pregnancy[95]

Having any of these risk factors increases the patient's risk of exacerbations even if they have few asthma symptoms

Other major independent risk factors for flare-ups (exacerbations)
- Ever intubated or in intensive care unit for asthma[96]
- ≥1 severe exacerbation in last 12 months[97]

Risk factors for developing fixed airflow limitation
- Preterm birth, low birth weight and greater infant weight gain[98]
- Lack of ICS treatment[99]
- Exposures: tobacco smoke;[100] noxious chemicals; occupational exposures[32]
- Low initial FEV_1;[101] chronic mucus hypersecretion;[100,101] sputum or blood eosinophilia[101]

Risk factors for medication side-effects
- *Systemic*: frequent OCS; long-term, high dose and/or potent ICS; also taking P450 inhibitors[132]
- *Local*: high-dose or potent ICS;[102,103] poor inhaler technique[104]

FEV_1: forced expiratory volume in 1 second; ICS: inhaled corticosteroid; OCS: oral corticosteroid; P450 inhibitors: cytochrome P450 inhibitors such as ritonavir, ketoconazole, itraconazole; SABA: short-acting beta₂-agonist.

*Excludes reliever taken before exercise. For children 6–11 years, also refer to Box 2-3, p.30. See Box 3-8, p.51 for specific risk reduction strategies.

[†]Independent' risk factors are those that are significant after adjustment for the level of symptom control. Poor symptom control and exacerbation risk should not be simply combined numerically, as they may have different causes and may need different treatment strategies.

Appendix 2: Individual sheet.

Group: controlled/uncontrolled

File no. :

Full name :

Current age :

***General :**

BMI (P/T^2) :Obese/overweight/normal weight

Passive smoking: yes/no

Active: yes/no

Socio-economic conditionsGood/average/poor Humidity at home: yes/no
Contact with pets: yes/no

***Clinical characteristics :**

Age of onset :

Age at diagnosis :

Duration of disease :

Allergic asthma: yes/no

Family atopy: yes/no (asthma, allergic rhinitis, atopic dermatitis, etc.)

Personal atopy: yes/no (allergic rhinitis, allergic conjunctivitis, atopic dermatitis)
Disease control during the last four weeks :

-number of bronchodilators used,

Symptoms/night-time awakenings (number of nights),

-Daytime symptoms (no. of days),

-Limitation of activity.
Disease profile over the last 12 months :

-number and severity of exacerbations,

-number of emergency consultations,

-number of hospital admissions,

-admission to intensive care for an asthma attack (yes/no),

-School absenteeism (no. of days),

-Limitation of physical activity (yes/no). Severity of asthma: mild/moderate/severe

***Psychological assessment:** teenagers/parents

***DEP :**

- > 80% of the theoretical

- :5 80% of the theoretical

***EFR :**

-normal,

obstructive ventilatory disorder: reversible/non-reversible.

***Biology:**

-Total IgE :

☐150 U/ml

<150 U/ml

-Level of eosinophils in the blood :

☐300/mm^3

<300/mm^3

***Current background treatment for asthma :**

(For each drug, specify: type/dose/route of administration)

-Inhaled corticosteroids (ICS).

Long-acting beta-2 mimetics (LABMs).

-Antileukotrienes.

***Inhalation technique :**

Metered-dose inhaler with or without inhalation chamber,

-Dry powder inhaler,

-boiling.

***treatment compliance:** good/poor

Appendix 3: BMI curve by age for boys.

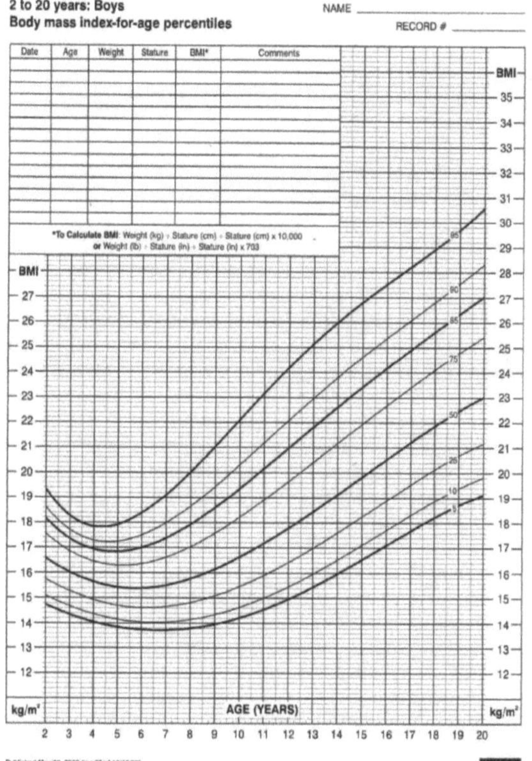

Appendix 3: BMI curve by age for girls.

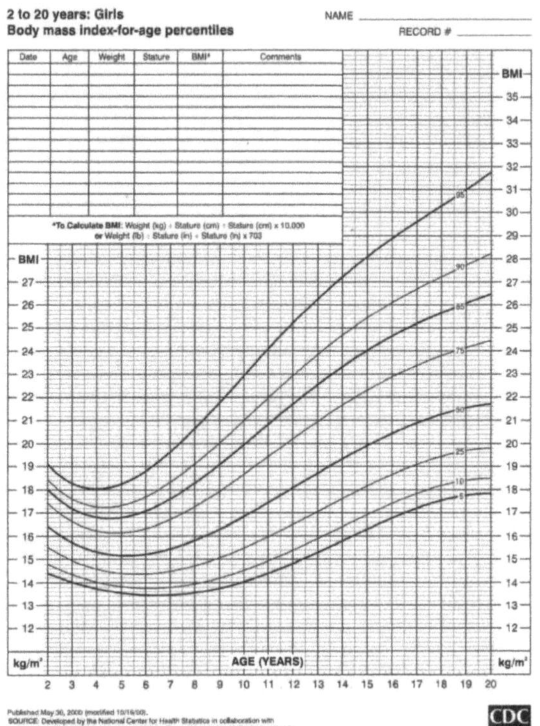

Appendix 4: GINA 2018 asthma severity stages.

Box 3-5. Stepwise approach to control symptoms and minimize future risk

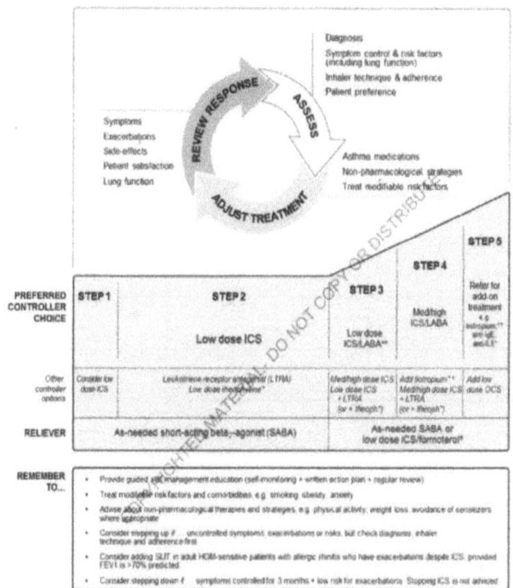

ICS: inhaled corticosteroids; LABA: long-acting beta2-agonist; med: medium dose; OCS: oral corticosteroids; SLIT: sublingual immunotherapy. See Box 3-6 (p 45) for low, medium and high doses of ICS for adults, adolescents and children 6–11 years. See Chapter 3 Part D (p 67) for management of exercise-induced bronchoconstriction.

* Not for children <12 years.
** For children 6–11 years, the preferred Step 3 treatment is medium dose ICS.
\# Low dose ICS/formoterol is the reliever medication for patients prescribed low dose budesonide/formoterol or low dose beclometasone/formoterol maintenance and reliever therapy.
† Tiotropium by mist inhaler is an add-on treatment for patients with a history of exacerbations; it is not indicated in children <12 years.

Appendix 5: theoretical EPD values children and adolescents (aged 5-18)

PEF (l/min)		
Height (cm)	Boys	Girls
100	106	105
105	132	132
110	159	158
115	185	185
120	212	211
125	238	237
130	265	264
135	291	290
140	318	317
145	344	343
150	370	369
155	397	396
160	423	422
165	450	449
170	476	475
175	503	501
180	529	528

FACTORS INFLUENCING ASTHMA CONTROL IN ADOLESCENTS

SUMMARY

Introduction:

Asthma is the most common chronic pathology among adolescents. Due to the physiological, psychological and behavioral changes inherent to adolescence, the management of this disease in this age group poses specific problems and constitutes an additional challenge. Improving the quality of life of adolescents with asthma essentially involves better asthma control. The objectives of our work were to clarify the clinical and progressive characteristics of asthma in adolescents and to identify the factors influencing the control of the disease.

Methods :

The study was descriptive, cross-sectional and retrospective involving 50 asthmatic adolescents. The patients were divided into a group of 28 controlled patients and a group of 22 uncontrolled patients.

Results:

There is a male predominance in both groups. Passive smoking was present in 48% of cases. Humidity in the home was present in 46% of cases. Asthma was allergic in 52.4% and 58.8% of controlled and uncontrolled patients respectively. The psychological evaluation interested only 14 adolescents (28%). Compliance was poor in 68.2% of uncontrolled patients. A moderate to severe decrease in PEF was noted in 42.9% of uncontrolled adolescents. All patients in the uncontrolled group were under treatment with inhaled corticosteroids with faulty inhalation technique in 16.7% of cases.

Factors for poor asthma control were:

* In the univariate study: the presence of humidity at home (OR=3.69), the reduction in peak expiratory flow in interictal (OR=5.5) and poor therapeutic compliance (OR=6.42) .

* In the multivariate study: poor therapeutic compliance (p=0.011).

Keywords :Asthma, adolescent, control

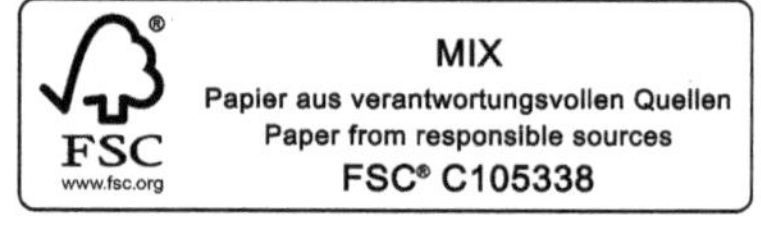

Printed by Books on Demand GmbH, Norderstedt / Germany